**THAMES AND HUDSON**

First published in Great Britain in 1974
First paperback edition 1990

Printed and bound in Great Britain by
Butler & Tanner Ltd, Frome and London

# CONTENTS

# PREFACE

The ever-widening response to this book since it was first published twenty years ago resulted in a number of later editions with new material added. This new material has been incorporated in the present volume, together with further new material and further changes. In effect, the book provided a basic source for learning about the life and work of the major "body-mind" innovator of the modern era. It also provided a standard text for teachers and students of the Alexander technique.

But a sizeable new audience has emerged, people without access to a teacher who seek to learn the technique directly from Alexander's own writings. He himself, the newcomers observe, had found his way with no outside assistance. Alexander in fact encouraged self-instruction. "You can do what I do," he said, "if you do what I did." In a late edition of one of his books, he even added a special preface addressed to "those who are anxious to teach themselves." In this context, he offered three pieces of advice. (1) Letters from these self-learners indicated that they were reading too hastily, and he warned them against "the habit of too quick reading in which understanding becomes dominated by speed." (2) From the very outset, neophytes had to realize that their old ways of doing and feeling could no longer be depended upon—"some of those who have complained of difficulty in trying to teach themselves may have overlooked this point." (3) For learn-it-yourself purposes, Alexander directed particular attention to the personal difficulties he himself had encountered and how he had freed himself from them.

In short, Alexander had no objection to people working on their own who accepted and kept in view his major points about the technique. "I would say, 'Go ahead,'" he stated bluntly; he promised a fundamental experience to anyone "with or without a teacher" who patiently applied the technique to ordinary living. At the same time, he emphasized that the whole process would go much faster with a teacher. (There were, of course, no more than a handful of teachers of the technique in his time. Even today, with the current proliferation of Alexander training programs, there are no more than a thousand instructors worldwide.)

The late Alexander authority, Frank Pierce Jones, also gave his blessing to self-learners, observing that "since the technique is nothing more than the application of experimental method to everyday behavior, there is no reason to delay the undertaking if a teacher is not available." Jones's practical suggestions for getting started are set forth on page 204. But enthusiasts would do well to read through these pages first, before embarking upon any self-help procedures.

Regardless of whether the reader intends to study and pursue the Alexander technique with or without a teacher, or simply wishes to find out about a unique and seminal genius of the twentieth century, Alexander's writings can hardly fail to prove stimulating and rewarding to all.

E.M.

# INTRODUCTION

"My experience may one day be recognized as a signpost directing the explorer to a country hitherto 'undiscovered,'" wrote the originator of the Alexander technique, describing the strange experience he underwent during the last decade of the nineteenth century. And so indeed has it turned out. The first thing about F. Matthias Alexander that strikes us today, more than a hundred years after his birth in Australia, is the remarkable sprawl of his influence on the current scene.

All over the western world people are engaged in doing most singular things with their bodies. Sometimes alone, sometimes in small intimate groups, and sometimes in massive orgy-like crowds, they have begun to disport themselves through a whole spectrum of bizarre physical activity. For better or for worse they have taken a sporting plunge into the mysterious waters of the "non-verbal."

There are, in fact, according to one catalog of the phenomenon, no fewer than sixty diverse and distinguishable forms of such performance to be observed on the landscape. And of these sixty or more goings-on, almost all are about as far as can possibly be imagined from anything that was in times past regarded as "physical training."

Large corporations confer upon select groups of executives and officials in their employ the privilege of attending seminars in the new body enlightenment. Universities, high schools, church groups, Y.M.C.A.'s, holiday resorts, department stores, schools of the theater and secret societies, along with the most certifiably wholesome community organizations, give regular courses or offer extension programs in it. And these may vary all the way from the continuously moving, serpentine gyrations of far-out, Far-Eastern calisthenics to the practically moveless, barely perceptible stirrings of home-grown Occidental hydro-psychotherapy.

Conservative newspapers and reasonably cautious magazines, which within living memory went out of their way to poke fun at the inclusion of such stuff in college curricula, now—under the respectful headings of "Education" and "Medicine"—pay unfailing and fastidious attention to it.

A conspicuous feature of the scene is the New Age version of a chain of old-style gymnasia once called human potential centers, and now called "holistic workshops," cropping up in Europe and America. "In several centers," explained Marshall McLuhan and George Leonard, two very early heralds of the movement, "they are working out techniques for awakening the body and senses..." From such experiments they predicted all people would one day find in themselves capacities for pleasure and fulfillment—beyond sex—that are barely hinted at in the present.

And as part of this widespread quest for a new fulfillment, the unique body-mind training which Matthias Alexander initiated during the period 1890 to 1900 has come into its own. Everywhere it attracts eager students from a generation which seems to comprehend immediately what it is all about. It is also perhaps the only method to be taken up by persons with a professional interest in their bodies—musicians, dancers, actors. Among the latter group, it ranks as a most precious secret of the contemporary theater. It is being tried as a promising educational tool in schools in England and America. It figures among the resources of physiotherapy available to the patients of great medical institutes in London and New York. Both *Vogue* and *Harper's Bazaar* proclaim the value of this training to the world of high fashion as well. American centers for the Alexander technique have been established country-wide to help meet the demand for teachers. In London, teachers have been trained uninterruptedly for many years, and in Denmark, Israel, France, Switzerland, Italy, Australia, South Africa and other countries, instruction in Alexander's technique has been offered for a long time now.

Indeed, Alexander begins to stand out as one of those innovators in the history of ideas and the development of feeling who are not put on the shelf after the recognition of legitimacy has once been granted their original concern. He has, most usefully, arrived right into the moment.

In his last years, he himself detected the first stirrings of the present excitement. "This, I believe," he wrote, "will now spread comparatively rapidly, and if it does, the work will soon come into its own..."

By "the work," of course, he meant the special body-mind technique which he had developed throughout his life. He always referred to it in that way. It was always "the work." And even those who followed him as teachers were, until quite recently, unable to come up with any more apposite name for it than "the Alexander technique."

"I see what you mean about a name," he once answered someone who wrote to complain of the lack. "That has been a matter of criticism for many a day. I reply: 'How can you name a thing that is so comprehensive?'" To the same correspondent he later amplified this difficulty in labeling "the work": "It is quite impossible for me to think of human manifestations as 'physical,' 'mental,' 'spiritual,' or in any separated form that might be named."

Today amid the agitated flutter which everywhere bestirs inquiry into the field of psychophysical education which Alexander opened up, his own discovery in it still holds a special appeal. It is simple, practical, precise. And amid the colorful array of body practices now being put forth, this one most notably requires neither the submergence nor the obliteration of our minds. What it uniquely offers, in fact, is nothing less than the prospect of a more rational control of our behavior.

Amid the engulfing sensoriness and mixed-media claimed by Marshall McLuhan for his "global village"; amid the revolutionary physicality voiced by ascendant groups in psychiatry, as well as by conspicuous ideologues of the body's resurrection; amid the wildly varied feely-centers and schools of the non-verbal proliferating on every hand; amid the kinetic partnership, joined by audience and cast alike, in current participatory drama; amid all these and many similar and characteristic features of our landscape, we are ready to approach with new heed what it was that he was trying to tell us, and even more, what it was that he was trying to do with the stream of people who came to him all those years of his life, when with a quality of single-mindedness bordering upon obsession, he pursued that solitary path which to so many of his contemporaries appeared a course of pure inexplicable goofiness.

And now that we understand what he was about, we can begin to see the man himself better. He was a peculiar genius who lacked the qualifications to establish scientifically the discovery which he made. Upon the development of that discovery, he bestowed in full measure the patience of genius. No longer need we form our image of him from wild conjectures about a sinister charlatan who unaccountably managed to bamboozle some of the most brilliant figures of our time. No longer need we speculate about what dire magnetism must have been exerted to dragoon men like Bernard Shaw, John Dewey and Aldous Huxley, among others, into his thrall. Alexander, it appears, had something genuine and valuable to teach.

Leonard Woolf, who could not fathom what the technique was about, but who visited him briefly and later brought Virginia Woolf to see him, once tried to clarify the ambiguous picture a little: "He was a remarkable man. He was a quack, but an honest, inspired quack... What was fascinating about him was that though fundamentally honest, he was at the same time fundamentally a quack." Woolf, who suffered from a lifelong tremor, believed the technique might have cured him if he had gone on with it: "I feel sure that he had hit upon a very important truth..." In the same way, in America where Alexander taught for extended periods, he was sometimes known as "the con man who really has the gold brick."

Even so hard-headed a type as John Dewey, one of the founding fathers of scientific philosophy and modern education, had to insist that "there is nothing esoteric in his teaching." Dewey considered it superior to psychoanalysis, and a necessary complement to that kind of treatment. Moreover, he pronounced it—a forgotten teaching of his—the necessary basis of all education. He himself had undergone an extraordinary rejuvenation after embarking upon "the work" at the age of 58, and continued to practice it to the end of his life. Dewey lived to a fit 93, and this vital longevity he always attributed to his Alexander training.

As a thinker, however, he took pains to deny that any personal indebtedness had gone into framing his estimate of the technique. For he had examined it objectively as well. "In affirming my convictions as to the scientific character of Mr. Alexander's discoveries and technique," Dewey protested, "I do so then not as one who experienced a 'cure,' but as one who has brought whatever intellectual capacity he has to the study of a problem."

Then, besides Dewey, there was that whole parade of other eminent personages who stepped forward to offer impressive testimony of what had been wrought for them. Heart trouble, arthritis, back pains, asthma, emphysema, bronchitis, even tuberculosis—a bewildering variety of human ailment and disorder, much of it chronic in nature, seems to have yielded quite miraculously to this method (though always, and most emphatically, its originator disclaimed anything "miraculous" about it). Take Aldous Huxley, for example, who after a lifetime spent in a state of acute physical disrepair, studied the technique and thereupon showed a surprising transformation. "His wife told me on Friday," wrote Alexander on February 3, 1936, "that they had dined with H. G. Wells the evening before, and that Wells had at once noticed the change in Huxley, and wanted to know the reason for it." The change had followed upon the two worst years of his life. In 1934 and 1935, Huxley had even begun to withdraw from people, finding any kind of social contact too much of a drain upon his physical and mental energies. To his customary afflictions were now added terrible depression and a chronic insomnia that made it all but impossible to work on the novel he was writing. After trying in vain to help himself by such means as gardening and yoga exercises, he began lessons with Alexander in October 1935—and apparently more than recovered. In describing how Alexander's method had liberated her husband's potentialities, Maria Huxley stated, "He has brought out, actively, all we, Aldous's best friends, know never came out either in the novels or with strangers."

With so many extravagant testimonials, it is no wonder there has been a suspicion, all these years, that the technique presents nothing more than

another historic example of the placebo-effect, that well-known phenomenon whereby cure is produced solely by faith in the instrument of cure.

A part of the atmosphere of mystery surrounding Alexander's reputation
derives from the self-legendizing propensity which he exhibited most of his
life. Though unquestionably evangelical about his work, when he came to
the "much needed spreading of the message," he was both conscientious and
rigorous about formulating it. About his personal history, however, he
sometimes indulged a robust tendency toward mythological splendor. In
addition, almost from the start he operated an impressive one-man public-
relations bureau on behalf of himself and the technique. Later, his students
and followers helped carry on this effective and—from the viewpoint of
reaching prospective students—doubtless necessary publicity job. The
result is that, today, simply to disentangle the bare facts of biographical
information requires a constant wariness in treating everything thus far
written and told about the man.

Frederick Matthias Alexander was born in Wynyard, a small town in
Northwest Tasmania, Australia, on January 20, 1869. His mother, with
whom he formed a special and lasting bond, was an excellent horsewoman.
She was possessed of a native talent for nursing, midwifery and other
medical services; and she employed this gift at the call of local doctors who
needed her. In cases of extreme urgency, she had been known to saddle up
and—no time to be lost fooling about with the gate!—leap over the paddock
fence as she rode off on her mission. Her son's profound instinctive empathy
with the moods and needs of his students, in later years, was sometimes
traced to this maternal heritage.

As a boy, Alexander went to school in Tasmania, but proved a most
awkward and difficult pupil because of his reluctance to take information on
trust and to submit to the usual routine. Eventually the schoolmaster, an
understanding Scotsman who had come to Australia for reasons of health,
saw the lad's father and arranged to give him private tutoring in the
evenings. (The unconventionality of his own early schooling did not, in later
life, make him any the more receptive to permissive trends in modern
education, which he strongly distrusted.) This was all the regular instruction Alexander ever received, but he did manage to win prizes and awards for
the school. Taking examinations came easily to him.

When it was time to leave school, his master wanted him to train for the
teaching profession, but he was just then offered a job with a tin mining
company. He accepted. Alexander later recalled that after he had broken the
news to the schoolmaster, they both sat in silence.

The truth was, he had no choice. Owing to family hardship, he as the
eldest child had to go out and earn. This was but the first imposition of a

financial load he was to carry from then on. Luckless, destitute or invincibly impoverished members of his family circle would always henceforth require his support. He remained head of the tribe. There would always be relatives, with children or without, who would be hard up and rely on his help. And the ensnarement of these responsibilities—descending now in early youth—would remain a permanent feature of his life and vocation. He would never be altogether free of such burdens. Thus at the age of 17, forswearing further education, he took off for the Mount Bischoff Tin Mining Company and went to work.

Despite his tender years, he performed a variety of functions, clerical, sales and bookkeeping, with considerable success in his new position. After three years, he had saved a good sum of money and left for Melbourne and a great spree which lasted as long as his funds. He dined on the choicest victuals and sipped vintage wines (he was forever a wine fancier, and a discriminating eater who relished good food), bought the best cut clothes he could find (he was forever a smart dresser, to whom elegant spats were a necessity), and since Sarah Bernhardt was then making her Australian tour, he went to see her twice a day.

From early childhood he had loved the theater, and already at the age of six began practicing the recitation that was then so much in vogue. This form of "declamatory thespianism" became his specialty. By the age of 19, he had gained a small reputation as a Shakespearian recitationist and had achieved professional status as an actor.

It was in Melbourne, after a succession of odd jobs, that he decided to go on the stage in earnest, both as recitationist and as actor.

And it was during this period that Alexander encountered the problem that was to occupy him through the next ten years and ultimately determine the direction of his life. This was a tendency for his voice to fail during recitals. When the trouble began, he went to doctors for help. The medical treatment, however, did little more than afford temporary relief. In time his condition became so aggravated that Alexander often could not bring himself to accept engagements when he felt uncertain of being able to get through a full evening of recitation. The climax was finally reached when he lost his voice halfway through an engagement which he regarded as particularly important to his career.

The following day, in the year 1888, he visited his doctor. It was for the last time. Thereafter he embarked upon a careful observation of how he was using himself physically in the act of public speaking. "Having the true scientific spirit and industry," his student Bernard Shaw later wrote, "he set himself to discover what it was that he was really doing to disable himself in this fashion by his efforts to produce the opposite result. In the end he found this out and a great deal more as well. He established not only the beginnings of a far-reaching science of the apparently involuntary movements we call reflexes, but a technique of correction and self-control which forms a substantial addition to our very slender resources in personal education."

The period of prolonged observation lasted for perhaps nine or ten years. At first, Alexander focused on what he might be doing that caused him to lose his voice. This scrutiny, done with the aid of mirrors, then gradually progressed far beyond the original problem. It widened to take in the whole psychophysical organism in activity. Of this trip beyond the looking glass, Alexander himself has provided a vivid and detailed account which need not therefore be repeated here.[1] In sum, however, what he found at the last was a very slight, all but imperceptible, yet seemingly inveterate accompaniment to every movement he made: a dismaying tendency to pull his head backwards and downwards. It was this involuntary constraint each time he undertook to declaim in public, or for that matter to perform the simplest physical act in private, which provided the key to his disability.

The prevention of it, he discovered, lay in a technique of physical reeducation based upon a certain dynamic relationship of the head, neck and torso (which will be discussed presently). Others before Alexander must have felt that relationship, but because it was a nonverbal, seemingly incommunicable experience, it had passed without formal record. What was extraordinary here was that the young Australian should have made it his mission in life to pinpoint the phenomenon, frame it in words and impart it to others.

"This story," writes Professor Niko Tinbergen, "of perceptiveness, of intelligence and of persistence, shown by a man without medical training, is one of the true epics of medical research and practice." In 1973, Tinbergen, awarded a Nobel Prize in physiology/medicine, and speaking as an ethologist, an authority on modes of attending animal behavior, chose the manner of Alexander's early investigation for special notice. "His research started some fifty years before the revival of ethology...yet his procedure was very similar to modern observational methods..." It was the old way of open-minded attention, of "watching and wondering" about behavior; a way not invented but brought back in the new animal studies. And "this basic scientific method," said Tinbergen, was what Alexander used through the years of the long quest leading to his discovery.

[1] See pages 139–160.

From the inexhaustible experimentation which he performed upon himself during this period, he also emerged with a bone-bred conviction that the mind and body were an inseparable whole: any attempt to treat one without the other was bound to fail. This would put him in opposition to the orthodox physical medicine of his day, as well as the unorthodox (osteopathy, chiropractic, rest cures, water cures, and other such forms of treatment). All of them, in his view, concentrated with lopsided emphasis on the body alone. Still later this organismic approach of his would set him apart from the burgeoning psychoanalytic movement which, in its exclusive preoccupation with factors of the psyche, he regarded as equally unbalanced.

Today, indeed, it is hard to conceive the dichotomy which then prevailed, not so much between body and mind, as between body and soul. Of this pair, the soul of course was superior; the body not merely inferior, but relegated to a position of extraordinary unworthiness and even degradation. The body, in the familiar parlance of that time, was simply a cross that had to be borne, a necessary evil. Thus before meeting Alexander, John Dewey (like many intellectuals) had been perfectly aware that he was inept in performing the physical tasks of existence. "Men are afraid," he later wrote, "without even being aware of their fear, to recognize the most wonderful of all the structures of the vast universe—the human body. They have been led to think that a serious notice and regard would somehow involve disloyalty to man's higher life." If he had to get up from a chair, or sit down, or pick up something he had dropped, he knew he would do it clumsily. Such awkwardness troubled him not at all: his aim was to get the physical business of life over with as quickly as possible so that he might get on to things that really mattered—like "thinking." From his study with Alexander, however, Dewey discovered that his own bodily activities were as appropriate a domain as any for the exercise of his highest abilities. He credited the technique therefore not only with having effected a marked improvement in his health, but also with having made him conscious of his total ignorance of a whole field of knowledge.

During the early years of his body-mind investigation, Alexander's voice began to improve, and on the basis of his preliminary findings he worked out a new method of breathing and of voice production. He did not at this stage, however, attach any larger significance to what he was doing.

After four or five years, he began teaching. By 1894, when Alexander was 25 years old, teaching had become his major career. The outline of what was later to become the "Alexander technique" was also by then beginning to take fairly definite form. It was during a six-month tour of recitals in Tasmania and New Zealand that Alexander began to glimpse a broader meaning in his work and what it might become. During the final three months in Auckland, he spent twelve hours a day at his teaching. When a tempting engagement to appear in America presented itself, Alexander turned it down. He embarked upon a strange risk.

For upon his return to Melbourne, his teaching took a new turn: breathing and voice production assumed a less important role than working with the technique.

Everywhere that he could find students, he taught. He gave lessons at the Roman Catholic college run by the Sacred Heart, a particularly well-known Order in Australia (and after classes was usually treated by the Superior to a warm comradely session of cognac and fine cigars). He traveled out to pupils in the mining towns of Ballarat and Bendigo, which he took in succession by train, arriving first at the one and teaching there, then continuing to the other, where he taught and spent the night, returning to Melbourne next day. While still with the tin mining company at Mount Bischoff, he had taught himself the violin, and sometimes to divert himself during these journeys as a peripatetic teacher, he would carry along his violin and play a few tunes.

A fairly renowned student of his Australian teaching days was the veteran actor Walter Bentley, who once said something Alexander afterwards liked to repeat. As a member of the Kean Company, Bentley had gone to Australia on tour and elected to stay there, performing in recitals, giving acting lessons and contriving a good livelihood. Impressed by the practical effectiveness of the technique, he one day proposed a spectacular plan by which the two men might join forces to exploit it. And that was when Bentley uttered those memorable words. "My boy," he told him, "I've been stamped on all my life, but now I'm a stamper, and by God I mean to stamp!" Alexander demurred. He did not fully understand what it was that he had, but he knew it was something not for exploitation but for future development.

His pupils now were mostly other voice-users (reciting was still in great favor), but before long, a number of them were patients sent to him by their doctors. Eventually, some members of the medical faculty at the University of Melbourne studied with him.

By the time Alexander moved to Sydney in 1899, his teaching was "basically one of changing and controlling reaction." While director of the Sydney Dramatic and Operatic Conservatorium during the next four years, he continued on that track. A well-known surgeon of the city, Dr. J. W. Stewart McKay, found that Alexander's technique was of benefit in certain gynecological cases, occasionally obviating the need for operations. Wholly on the basis of McKay's encouragement Alexander decided he would go to London to make his technique known. During the year preceding his departure, he busied himself with a theatrical group composed of his own pupils, with whom he presented thirty performances each of *Hamlet* and of *The Merchant of Venice,* first in Sydney and then on tour. On April 13, 1904, at the age of 34, he sailed for London.

During the long ocean journey from Australia, he was occupied with writing the first draft of a book which would explain his technique. But he threw the pages into the sea just before the boat reached port. The four books[1] he would ultimately publish, together with the constant alterations and modifications he made in them through a long sequence of revised editions, were to be assembled only as the adjunct and embellishment of a lifetime spent in practical teaching. In the writing of them he would determinedly try to steer clear of all medical and psychological jargon, irritating the professionals by his simplistic avoidance of technical terms. His books are by no means formal compositions. Devoid of grace, style or shape, they are the earnest patching together of observation and experience by a unique authority who had never received any real instruction in the mechanics of writing.[2] They were meant to provide a source of original material on a new subject: that they do.

Next to "the work," horse racing was the major passion of Alexander's life. It started when he was a youngster Down Under, where everyone went to the races and everyone had some loose change to back a favorite nag. Through the rest of his days he never left off, and continued avidly to play the horses. In prosperous years after he became established, he maintained a number of betting accounts under different names. At one time, he is reported to have placed a bet every half hour of each working day. A handyman, and afterwards a teaching assistant, were trained to place these bets for him when he was occupied giving lessons. At 16 Ashley Place, the famous headquarters which he set up in London, an extra telephone had to be installed whenever he was visited by his brother, who shared a similar penchant for the track. It was needed to accommodate the overload of betting calls that were being made.

It was this passion which got Alexander off to a rousing start when he first arrived in London. He had pondered whether he could afford the journey, since there were female relatives, including his mother, who were in part dependent upon him financially. Mounting a tram one day, he sat next to a bookmaker of his acquaintance. The bookie asked if he might be interested in placing a bet that would pay one-hundred-fifty to one.

---

[1] See Bibliographic Note pages xlvii-xlviii.
[2] The reader might therefore be advised to begin with the prefaces by Dewey (Appendix I).

Alexander said indeed he would, placed a £5 bet, and won £750. His London career was off and running.

London was always agreeable, especially during the spring. He met with early recognition there which proved highly lucrative as well. Lessons with "F.M." (his familiar name) were expensive. Many of those who met his price whether they could afford to or not were in sadly ailing or in decrepit condition. He called them the "old crocks," in contradistinction to the regulars who came in quest of well-being or self-realization. Those who could not produce the full amount of his fees were the "cheap people." He later referred them to his assistants for lessons. With youngsters, "F.M." was unequaled, freely entering the world of childhood as teacher and accomplice. He liked to play.

Supple and slim, with a remarkable symmetry of physique, he bore no resemblance to the typical muscle man who then instructed in physical culture. In a field largely monopolized by mesomorphs, he was a stray. The thing one remembered most about him, apart from the really incredible— and sometimes jarring—dynamism of the man, was the startling wide-awakeness of the eyes looking out from the oval face.

Actors and actresses flocked to learn the technique, as they do today. The great Sir Henry Irving became an ardent student. Others through the years included Lily Brayton, Viola Tree, Constance Collier, Oscar Asche, Lily Langtry and Matheson Lang. (Later still came the film stars.) In the early days he often went, by hansom or taxi, to work with the stars in their dressing rooms just before they were called on stage. At one point, he was traveling to as many as five different theaters before curtain-raising time.

From a number of prominent London physicians, he received encouraging support, particularly from Dr. R. H. Scanes Spicer, an elderly enthusiast who sent him patients. It was the true beginning of Alexander's endless, tantalizing love-hate relationship with the medical profession: after six years he published "A Protest" against Dr. Spicer for claiming too much of the technique as his own discovery.

As a consequence of World War I, with everyone caught up in service or patriotic effort, the flow of students all but stopped. Like an artist denied paint and canvas, or a chemist deprived of a laboratory, Alexander lacked the human material he needed for "the work" and departed for America in search of new pupils. In the first month of the war, he sailed for New York, and by the end of September 1914, he was teaching nine hours a day.

It was the start of what was ultimately to develop into an intercontinental mission. Besides John Dewey, other influential figures in America like Lewis Mumford, Waldo Frank, Leo Stein and James Harvey Robinson (not to mention J. B. Duke, the tobacco magnate), were all to become interested in the technique. Professor Robinson in 1919 published in the *Atlantic Monthly* a glowing article about it, entitled "The Philosopher's Stone." The piece attracted widespread attention.

The reception in America was not without its dark side, however. Randolph Bourne, the brilliant radical writer, had serious reservations not about the efficacy of the method but about its purported bearing on the future of humanity, and fairly early, detected a flavor of cultism in the commotion that was being made. In England as well, complaints on this score began to be heard. Many a convinced initiate was able to continue with the technique only by deliberately ignoring the worshipful aura which hovered about the person of its progenitor.

And most gracefully, most deftly, but nonetheless ruthlessly, the master began to exploit the energies of his more devoted pupils. In grave and measured language, he expounded the necessity of attending to "means" rather than to "ends": meanwhile his dutiful followers hustled about and managed to obtain the personal "ends" he desired. While he virtuously maintained a state of composed concentration upon the "means-whereby," more often than not it was their strenuous "endgaining" that got him the results he wanted. (To procure him a large shipment of the tea he liked, they once had to work a solid couple of years, while stringent British rationing was in effect; students influential in government on both sides of the Atlantic—Christian Herter in America, and Sir Stafford Cripps in England—were also called upon to lend a hand in cutting the red tape involved in this tedious entanglement.) The radical "ends-means" dichotomy, a philosophically dubious and recurrent theme in Alexander, remained a permanent influence upon the thinking of such students as Aldous Huxley, who based and titled a book upon it, and continued to rely upon the sharp artificial distinction to the end of his writing.[1]

After the war, and until 1924, Alexander still taught quite regularly in New York during the months from November to April. In America it was, in fact, considered very social during the twenties to study with "F.M." or with "A.R.," For his brother, Albert Redden Alexander, whom he had trained in Australia, maintained a Boston outpost until his death in 1947. Assistant teachers on occasion also came to America with "F.M." But except for his confidence in "A.R." he remained both cavalier and variable in estimating the competency of his teachers, no matter how loyal or how long trained. In fostering and developing a consistent program for the training of teachers, he was likewise agonizingly undependable. There were times when

---

[1] See however pages xxxvi-xxxvii for the usefulness of this terminology in the technique itself.

he appeared to regard the technique as simply a matter of "doing his own thing."

Unknown to his closest associates, Alexander during this period of his intercontinental mission had assumed the proud and deliberate status of "undischarged bankrupt." It had nothing to do with anything so crass as a lack of money: it was a matter of principle. Before his original journey to America, he had purchased a car which would not go. The dealers offered no satisfaction and he refused to pay till they did. While he was overseas, they took him to court. Afterwards they put the account in the hands of a collection agency. It was not to be borne. That they would deal with him so unscrupulously in the first place, that they would then take legal action in his absence when he had no opportunity of defending himself, and that they would then put the matter in the hands of a third party who had nothing whatever to do with it—there was no other redress open to him: he refused to pay and allowed himself to be made a bankrupt.

When Alexander finally appeared in court, this straightforward presentation of his case must have reached a sympathetic receiver. For he was pronounced an "undischarged bankrupt" who was nonetheless granted so many special exemptions as to emerge in a remarkably undismantled state of bankruptcy. He could maintain a bank account, obtain goods on credit, and otherwise carry on quite as comfortably as before, except of course that his new status foreclosed the possibility of ever joining a club. Since Alexander had no wish to join any club, he never afterwards did anything to alter the benign judgment. (Sometime after World War II, however, an old friend, fearing the effects of Alexander's unique financial condition upon the formation of a teachers' society, bought the debt at a nominal sum from the collection agency, and tore it up.)

The whole episode revealed Alexander once again as the incongruous blend he had become: half London dandy, the city sophisticate who, attuned to the more subtle refinements of living, collected Sheffield Plate in Pimlico; half blunt Aussie, still the rough lad who had gone to work in the tin mining company so sadly, "because with deep regret I finished the way of life I had enjoyed up to that time, the outdoor experience in the fields, the sea and the beaches."

Alexander married Edith Page, an Australian actress, in 1920. Three years later he bought a house and twenty acres at Bexley, Kent. Mrs. Alexander, theatrical, estranged and remote, lived a separate life of personal embitterment. Not long after their marriage she had suffered a seizure, or type of stroke. Half her face was paralyzed, the muscles affected in some manner. From having been an exceptionally beautiful woman, she now looked upon herself as hideous. She took up the life of a recluse, established her own residence and was afterwards tended until her death in 1938 by their adopted daughter. For Alexander it remained a particular sorrow that he, who had been able to do so much to help so many, could do nothing at all for the person nearest him. Till the day she died, he experienced a tender concern for her and continued to visit on weekends. His wife became fiercely antagonistic to "the work," and even decreed that he must never give lessons to their daughter. In later years, a mistress (of Australian background) and a natural son became accepted and uncommented-upon members of his household. To the public, his companion, in accordance with Victorian custom, appeared to be no more than housekeeper and efficient manager of school premises.

In 1924, Alexander established a school for children, from the ages of three to eight, at his teaching quarters in London. (The "little school" he called it.) It was later endorsed through a trust fund by the Earl of Lytton, former Viceroy of India, another of his students. The technique also expanded at an unexpected rate in South Africa through the efforts of an exceptionally venturesome teacher who carried "the work" there in 1935. (One of her contacts, Dr. Raymond A. Dart, the distinguished anthropologist who was Professor of Anatomy at the University of Witwatersrand, in Johannesburg, taught himself the technique and subsequently published three articles inspired by it.) Alexander at the time—during the two years from 1933 to 1935—was busy putting on performances of *Hamlet* at the Old Vic and of *The Merchant of Venice* at Sadler's Wells. It was a repeat of what he had done long before in Sydney, and again the cast was made up of himself and his pupils. He, needless to say, took the juicy role of Shylock himself. Next to "the work" and playing the horses, a balked desire to appear on the stage may have been his dominant passion.

This histrionic inclination discomfited some advocates of the technique. Others were completely put off by it. A. M. Ludovici, for example, in his autobiography, testifies to the good results of his lessons: "It is impossible fully to describe the benefits both in health and *joie de vivre* which I owed, and still owe, to this radical alteration in my physique; for although nothing could of course correct all my constitutional failings, I was a changed man... It has certainly prolonged my life." At first, however, Ludovici had almost decided against studying with Alexander: "I found his incessant accompanying patter rather distracting, and was not impressed by its purport. He would break off from time to time and, in a deep and attractive voice, declaim a passage from Byron or Shakespeare which seemed to me to bear little relevancy to the matter in hand. Altogether, I thought him too reminiscent of a showman, and there and then decided to have nothing to do with him." (After he had reversed his opinion he wrote a book about him.)

On a less elevated plane of performance, though, Alexander could be nothing short of captivating. With his slightly exaggerated gestures, his authentic mannerisms, his salty way of saying the words, he conquered all within range when he recounted his old stories from Down Under. He was inimitable. "Many of us felt after hearing him recite his Australian tales," wrote the American teacher Lulie Westfeldt in her memoir, "that he could have made a fortune any day as a comedian. I, for one, never doubted it. Where his own particular brand of humor was concerned, he was a great artist and irresistible."

With the outbreak of World War II, the children's school, accompanied by Alexander and three teachers, was evacuated to America, and there reestablished at the Whitney Homestead in Stowe, Massachusetts, under the auspices of the Unitarian Association of America. The estate was turned over to him rent-free for this purpose, and some American children joined the school. Alexander was now 71 years old and, as before, the outbreak of war virtually put a stop to the flow of students in England.

He returned to England in May 1943, and the next year became enmeshed in a complex series of legal proceedings. He had been affronted by a scathing attack upon his work published in South Africa by Dr. Ernst Jokl, a physical education officer of the government there, and unable to obtain either the withdrawal of offending statements, or the possibility of full-scale refutation in the official journal which carried them, he decided to bring suit for libel. The case expanded and extended until it finally came to trial in Johannesburg in 1948. Alexander won the case and the judgment in his favor was subsequently confirmed, the following year, by the Supreme Court of Appeal. The affair, however, had proved an enormous drain on time, energy and money. Two Nobel laureates in physiology/medicine, E.D. Adrian and Sir Henry Dale, had testified against some of the claims made for the technique, which Dale labeled "intensely dangerous quackery" that ought to be made "criminal." The judge's decision, apart from the winning legalities that pertained to libel, had provided a shadowed victory since it concurred with the testimony of the two Nobel witnesses that "in its claims to cure, the system constitutes dangerous quackery."

It was during the period of the libel action, in late 1947, that Alexander had a fall which displaced one rib and bruised several others. Within a week of the accident, he suffered a stroke and lost the use of his left arm and leg. The left side of his face was also paralyzed, as can be seen in a portrait painted at the time. He was now 79, but the following year he was again giving lessons: he had recovered a substantial use of his arm and leg, and the paralysis in his face was barely noticeable. A crude film of him taken thereafter reveals him as still lithe and youthful in movement. We see him showing off a bit as he casually brings one leg over a chair and back to the floor. Then, for some reason dissatisfied with that performance, he repeats the gesture, leg effortlessly uplifted over the chair and down again. It was one of the feats with which he liked to entertain students.

There were still almost eight active years ahead of him. He continued to teach to within days of the end, at the age of 86. Returning from a good afternoon at the races, followed by a splendid dinner of lobster, he was taken by a sudden chill. Confined to his bed thereafter, he asked that a radio be brought to his room so that he might keep abreast of racing results. Sitting up against pillows, he wrote letters, signed cheques and conducted necessary business.

During these last few days, his physician had asked a young local doctor to keep an eye on him. The brisk young man bustled into Alexander's room, saying, "Well, how are we today?" The patient, in extremely acid tones, replied, "I am very well indeed, thank you." All his life, Alexander had frowned upon the practice of asking anyone "How are you today?" In the first place, he was careful to explain, people do not *know* how they are. In the next place, getting them to *think* about it is a wrong stimulus, very bad for them. This form of greeting had always annoyed him, always irritated him: it was rude. On his deathbed he still refused to countenance it.

He died on October 10, 1955.

What was the significance of "the work"? What was it all about and what was Alexander trying to do? Just what was he, and now those who teach his method, the new Alexandrians, trying to tell us about the use of the self?

To begin with, what do they mean by the use of the self? The answer lies in how you move, how you stand, how you sit; your bearing—in short, the total scope of your activity. The static word "posture" will not do. The word may serve very well to describe the condition of your stance as you enter a room or the position you assume as you stand poised at the head of a staircase. But once you have made your entrance or the very second you begin to descend any staircase, you are again caught up in movement. And your old habits will reappear immediately if their absence was based on nothing more than that transient "holding-in" commonly called posture.

Even the posture professionals—the marching line at the military academy or the prancing chorus line at Radio City—have to let go in ordinary life. Beyond the parade ground and the proscenium, both the cadets and the Rockettes must relinquish their strenuously maintained (and fatiguing) body attitudes. For you cannot attain a correct posture and then cling to it throughout all your subsequent activity. That would be like transporting a statue from place to place and propping it about, here and there, in various juxtapositions. Getting up, sitting down, walking, standing, opening and closing drawers, entering or leaving cars, dressing and undressing, shutting windows, reaching for a pencil, unscrewing the top of a mayonnaise jar: *all* our usual activities, from the most strenuous to the least effortful, involve us in *complicated patterns of movement and rest which, for better or worse, constitute our particular use of ourselves.*

"Mr. Alexander has done a service to the subject," wrote Sir Charles Sherrington, the Nobel-prize physiologist, "by insistently treating each act as involving the whole integrated individual, the whole psychophysical man. To take a step is an affair not of this or that limb solely but of the total neuromuscular activity of the moment—not least of the head and neck."

But how then do we acquire a better use of ourselves, and with it an improved approach to the activities of living? If behavior is mainly movement, what is the prerequisite of good movement? As early as 1907, Alexander identified this prerequisite with the greatest lengthening of the spine possible in whatever we may be doing. It was this vertebral lengthening in activity which he then called "the true and primary movement in each and every act." (A quarter of a century later, he began applying to it the much less satisfactory term "primary control.")

About the complex neuromuscular mechanisms which regulate this spinal lengthening, especially as involved in the combined functioning of reflex and voluntary movement, Alexander was never too clear. But about what was practically required to maintain it flexibly throughout any and every form of movement, he had no doubts at all. This he knew from direct experience. It was maintained by a special head-neck-torso relationship which he could feel, and which seemed to have three main characteristics.

To describe, even to prescribe, this three-fold pattern is deceptively simple:

(1) Let the neck be free (which means merely to see that you do not increase the muscle tension of the neck in any act).
(2) Let the head go forward and up (which means merely to see that you do not tense the neck muscles by pulling the head back or down in any act).
(3) Let the torso lengthen and widen out (which means merely to see that you do not shorten and narrow the back by arching the spine).

But these are instructions which are no instructions at all. They cannot even be carried out literally. Taken together, they point to one unified sensation, a single felt experience that seems to permit or expedite the desirable elongation of the spine which constitutes "the true and primary movement in each and every act." Or as Alexander enigmatically summarized these three directions: "All together one after another."

Since this is the way in which we are habitually to make use of ourselves, the Alexandrians reject all forms of physical manipulation as a means of achieving it. A golfer, let us say, might find through physical manipulation, temporary relief from the painful strains caused by a faulty swing. If his pain is not to recur, however, the error in his swing must be eliminated.

The Alexandrians likewise reject corrective exercise as a path to good use of the self. For here they agree with the nursery rhyme that so usefully reminds us, "There was a crooked man who walked a crooked mile." That is to say, if we comport ourselves in a manner that is all wrong, any exercise we engage in to correct this condition is likely to be carried out in a manner that is all wrong too. It will thus fail to correct anything. Alexander's lifelong running criticism of sports, calisthenics and athleticism in general, still makes cogent reading,[1] and some of his major points are reflected in the valuable reforms now being introduced in these conventional approaches to physical education. More and more, even in simple programs of aerobics, attention is paid to how they are carried out.

The main problem, really, as the Alexandrians see it, is that we have all become so accustomed to our usual way of doing things that it "feels right" and reliable to us. No matter how poorly coordinated we may be, it "feels right." So any more efficient or better way of doing things is bound to "feel wrong" and unreliable. How then may we ever learn to conduct ourselves in a new way that will "feel wrong" in the beginning?

Obviously words can be of small help to the teacher who would initiate such a change in our customary functioning. The problem here goes far beyond the usual difficulty with using words to teach anything—that is, our familiar disposition to accept language as language, without transforming it into the actuality of conduct or deportment. In an anecdote in his *Journals,* the Danish theologian Kierkegaard has neatly encapsulated this common failure: a raw recruit is being instructed by a corporal in the bearing and behavior of a soldier. "You must hold yourself erect in the ranks," says the corporal. "Aye, aye, I understand that," says the recruit. The corporal continues: "And you must not talk while under arms." The recruit: "Oh, is that so; well, I am glad you have told me, so that now I know about it." "What the devil," says the corporal, "did I not tell you to keep your mouth shut!" "Aye, but do not be angry with me; now that I understand it I shall be sure to remember it."

[1] See pages 109–113.

Beyond this normal resistance to verbal instruction, however, Alexander had to contend with another, more basic problem, which was inherent in what he was attempting. His task was like sending a kiss by messenger. The experience he sought to impart was one which by its very nature eludes utterance. As is usually pointed out, you cannot describe "blue" to a man who has never seen the color blue. How then do you convey a new feeling, a new pattern of physical sensation, to a man who has never known it? For what Alexander sought to teach in his lessons was not, as may at first appear, the concerted positioning of certain body segments. Rather, the technique involves a faculty that we all possess but frequently overlook because it is not one of the so-called "five senses" listed by Aristotle.

Almost everyone, however, knows a little something about the "kinesthetic sense," or the "muscle sense" as it is sometimes incorrectly called. In fact its sense organs are to be found not only in the muscles but in the tendons and joint membranes as well. It is by means of this sense, for example, that when our eyes are closed we continue to be aware of the position of every part of our body. It is from this sense that we derive knowledge of the gestures we make and of the pressures or tensions anywhere in our body. We use it to assess the range and force of our movements, and also in adapting ourselves to the weight of anything we lift.

This "crown of the senses," hardly mentioned any more in the fever of national physical fitness campaigns, was not always omitted from consideration in earlier drives for public health. Taking part in one such effort in 1920, the sophisticated New England medical educator, Dr. George V. N. Dearborn, crusaded for recognition of the prominent place the kinesthetic sense holds in the life of every individual. "The warp of the sensation-fabric—the personality's dynamic index of its body," was his strong definition of it.

The importance of this sense in a man's life is unfortunately not diminished by his ignorance of it, said Dearborn. He could only feel pity for a man, however excellent his objective mind, who has never developed so as to become conscious of this world of submerged sensation. To him such a person must remain always "a clumsy boor, materialistic by nature, loath to become familiar with himself."

One trouble, as Dr. Dearborn pointed out, is that the too dominant sense experiences of light and color and sound drown this subtler experience, sometimes so completely that many intelligent adults go through life "wholly ignorant even of the essential existence of these warp threads in the fabric of our conscious life."

And it is this "crown of the senses" which gives us the key to understanding the technique developed by Alexander. His original search for the source of his recitation difficulties may indeed have begun with the visual, as he perseveringly scrutinized the three mirrors with which he had surrounded himself. But that search ultimately extended itself, through the next several years, to the kinesthetic. He did not establish any control over his problem until he could kinesthetically perceive that he was about to pull his head back and down each time before commencing to declaim. Without this kind of felt knowledge, as a preliminary, any attempt to bring about lasting reform in the use he was making of himself would have proved impossible. "You can do what I do," Alexander liked to say, "if you do what I did."

One of his earliest publications was a pamphlet in 1908 entitled "Re-education of the Kinesthetic System (Sensory Appreciation of Muscular Movement) Concerned with the Development of Robust Physical Well-being." As Bernard Shaw remarked, "Alexander calls upon the world to witness a change so small and so subtle that only he can see it." For we learn from this technique a kinesthetic way of adapting ourselves to our environment, no matter what we may be doing. We apply ourselves, henceforth, by means of a new experience involving head, neck and trunk. We proceed with a fresh overall sensation of lightness and ease in the handling of our bodies.

Initially, Alexander had attempted—in words, futile words—to teach the new feeling by *telling* his pupils how to attain it. Visitors to his first headquarters in London could observe the two brothers, "F.M." and "A.R.," each with a single pupil and at opposite ends of the studio, shouting their disparate and desperate verbal instructions at the two victims. All patience with language had been exhausted.

In the end, "whereof one cannot speak, thereof one must be silent," as the Austrian philosopher Wittgenstein was to write years later. But instead of relying upon words in situations whereof one cannot speak, might there not be some other form of communication? Might it not be possible to impart one's message in some other way? In meeting and solving this problem, Alexander developed a means for conveying kinesthetic experience—which is perhaps the most valuable part of his work. He became the true father in Western culture of what Aldous Huxley called the "non-verbal humanities."

Those who teach the Alexander technique today follow the ingenious form of instruction which he evolved. It is an enterprise requiring the closest cooperation between student and teacher.

First, what is required of the student? During lessons he or she, when called upon to perform any given activity, must simply refuse to do anything at all. Stand? Sit? Walk? He simply refuses each time to do anything. This does not mean that he remains in a state of inert collapse. For one thing, he works consciously at refusing those involuntary preparations—sometimes called "sets"—that he always, in the past, made before going into any such acts. It is the subtle, taken-for-granted habits of getting ready for every move that must be revealed and prevented. (Lifting a full suitcase that turns out to be empty, or stepping to an extra stair that does not happen to be at the top of the staircase, we are sometimes made acurely aware of these unconscious habits of readiness.)

The reader of this page is now asked to stand up for a moment .... Stop! Before even starting to rise from your sofa or chair, did you perhaps begin to forshorten the muscles at the back of your neck? If so, that constitutes a part of your particular "set," or involuntary preparation for getting up. It is also an example of the kind of thing that you would gradually learn to prevent during lessons.

With this special form of cooperation from the student, the teacher then "stands" him, "sits" him, "walks" him, encouraging the desired head-neck-torso relationship throughout the process. To the degree to which the student does not intrude any of his old habits, he allows the teacher's manual guidance to give him, over and over again, a new sensory experience of these common acts. And in his new movements, which might be called "reflex facilitated"[1] rather than active or passive, there occurs a redistribution of postural tone. Finally, sitting, standing, walking *like this* —or engaging in no matter what activity *like this*—begins to "feel right." His neck feels free, his head feels as if it is going forward and up, and his torso feels as if it is lengthening and fanning out toward the shoulders. Between lessons, he will continue saying "no" to his old movements, actively permitting their replacement by the new ones acquired during lessons.

Lessons in the technique form a gradual process with a fascination of its own. The end result is that, in time, the special requisite head-neck-torso pattern is established and continues as the major feature in all of our activities. Nothing static: nothing "postural." Head, neck and torso—like every other part of the body—are freely and independently movable at all times. There persists, however, a certain dynamic relationship among them. And it is this relationship, presumably, which allows the greatest lengthening of the spine as "the true and primary movement in each and every act."

---

[1] For the important topic of anti-gravity reflexes, see Appendix III. The anatomical and physiological explanations put forward to account for the new facts of space medicine (for example, that skylab astronauts living without the effects of gravity gain inches in height and lose inches around the waist) are interesting in the present context.

There are an overall flexibility and tonic ease of movement, greater freedom in the action of the eyes, less tension in the jaws, more relaxation in the tongue and throat, and deeper breathing because of the effect of the new alignment on the diaphragm. There are also a sense of weightlessness and a diminution of the effort previously thought necessary to move one's limbs. Activity is now more free and flowing—no longer jerky and heavy with strain.

This lighter-than-air effect must not, at all costs—as Alexander insisted—be confused with what is usually meant by "relaxation." John Dewey, in a letter, mentioned "Alexander's point that when people are told to relax, they do so at one locus and tense themselves at another place." This tendency, Dewey believed, might be tested objectively.

More importantly, however, Alexander was appalled by the customary approach to the problem. To relax, in his meaning of the word, does not mean that you should become a bag of bones. If one observes a cat or dog at rest, one will see what true relaxation is: the dog and cat are completely relaxed, yet they are still capable of making sudden and definite movements. Alexander deplored the lack of muscular tone in students who, in later years, came to him after having undergone the new relaxation training. The purpose of his technique, as he saw it, was not to get rid of tensions, but to reorganize them into a source of energy and satisfaction.

The question of breathing likewise receives unique emphasis in his work. Alexander, from the very start of his career, opposed the schools of "deep breathing" then in vogue. He was interested, rather, in coaxing an awareness of breathing as it supports movement, and of movement as it reinforces breathing. The possibilities of orchestration between the two, in activity, are practically infinite. "We never talk about breathing," Alexander once cryptically informed a pupil, thus expressing his deep concern with it only as manifest in the precise exigencies of doing: it was to be seen only as a function of using oneself properly.

After all, one never has to worry about whether or not breathing is going on. The question is whether it is free or forced. If it is forced, said Alexander, the point is not to deliberately sniff or suck in the air. Always, in "the work," you simply allow your breathing to take place in accord with your expanding, decreasing, ever-changing needs as you move about—or remain still—in many different ways. The ribs are to expand naturally, and the respiration is to be felt even in one's back, exhalation rather than inhalation being the only point of interest.

The technique's approach to the problem of physical and mental health is an indirect one. In a letter to the *British Medical Journal,* Alexander wrote, "I have expressly dissociated myself from any idea of producing 'cures,' or giving 'treatment.'" He had been deservedly rapped over the knuckles by a previous correspondent to the *Journal* because there are indeed passages in his writings where he cannot resist sounding like the super-physician who knows how to outdoctor the doctors. But these are nothing more than crowing lapses of self-gratulation. He did know better. For many years, medical men had been sending their patients to him solely because of his experience in examining conditions of use, and in estimating the influence of such conditions upon functioning. "I would say at once," wrote Alexander in one book, "that I do not receive these cases as patients, but as pupils, inasmuch as I am not interested in disease or defects apart from their association with harmful conditions of use and functioning." The revised version of his first book significantly replaces the incautious word "patient" with the word "pupil."

This point is basic, since no attempt is ever made by Alexander teachers to treat a particular symptom—which they are not in any case qualified to do. They are concerned rather with establishing the positive conditions for health. In those cases where the techniques may be called upon by medical men, a present-day teacher has compared the method with tidying up an untidy room in order to find a missing object rather than searching for it directly. "The indirect way," he writes, "may take a little longer, but it is more certain, will render further losses less likely, and will have accomplished something useful even if the missing object remains unfound. Also it may happen that something lost long since and which has been forgotten may turn up. It has, too, the further important advantage that one will at last become fully aware of the contents of the room in a way that one had not been before." This is something of a parallel with the method used, for "not only do symptoms disappear in the process which have resisted more direct methods but also there is less likelihood of recurrence, and even if the symptoms persist, the person is still much better off at the end." So too, he points out, may unexpected and unlooked-for benefits occur, like the disappearance of headaches or the feeling of greater self-confidence or an improvement in concentration. To complete the parallel with the tidied-up room, he mentions the greater awareness of the physical self which is obtained. For some people this may prove one of the most valuable gains derived from their lessons: it helps offset the tendency to treat the body as a machine to be driven, rather than as a living thing entitled to respect in its own right.

Where Alexander teachers are unavailable, groups of prospective students can sometimes organize and locate a teacher willing to travel to their vicinity for a brief spell.

There is no definite number of lessons prescribed for attaining results. The best thing is for students to use their own judgment, both with respect to length of instruction and funds available to cover the cost. After that they may continue longer with their teacher, if they can make use of further assistance and can afford to pay for it. Or they may decide to work on their own, returning at future intervals for more lessons as needed. But it is important not to be abject about this question, not to accept any certain standardized number of lessons as requisite for one and all who would learn.

The old-fashioned stock estimate used to range from six to twenty or thirty consecutive lessons, depending on how badly a student might be out of kilter. For some students, however, only intermittent lessons may be possible. In one legendary instance a single lesson sufficed. Again, there are those rare persons with a coordination which seemingly has nothing more to gain from any form of instruction. The boxer Muhammad Ali in his prime inspired this kind of awe, at first sight, in one teacher: "He drifted about the ring like a piece of blown thistledown, always in balance and always ready to move or strike."

Learning the technique, of course, is not a once-and-for-all thing, but is meant to continue beyond lessons as a development process on one's own, with further growth and proficiency. Within the context of everyday life it is easy to lapse: when you enter a cab, for example. You may simply drop out of all physicality and, with utter lack of perception, merely persist in a cerebral haze or a state of dull blankness towards your surroundings until the time you are delivered at your destination.

The true objective of lessons is to launch a person upon a course of self-discovery which leads to increased awareness and control: the lessons are not a conditioning procedure. Notwithstanding Alexander's credo of universal salvation, the technique is simply not for everyone—once past childhood—though there seems to be no way at all of predicting who will or will not be able to learn it. There is an enormous variation from person to person in "use" and in reliability of feeling. (Lawyers and mathematicians Alexander lumped together at the bottom of the scale.) W.C. Fields's classic advice probably applies here: "If at first you don't succeed, try, try again. Then quit. No use being a damn fool about it ..." To this might be added the further advice: or try another teacher.

The difficulties in estimating both the number of lessons required, and their probable effectiveness, may derive in part from the lack of any coherent theory as to how and when humans went awry in the use of themselves.

Alexander attributed our predicament to the increased and ever-changing demands which civilization places upon us. The eminent American biologist George E. Coghill, to whom he gave lessons in Florida and who supported "the work," offered him some corroboration for the idea. Coghill after 1900 had begun the first systematic observation of embryonic behavior. The most suitable subject for such investigation, it turned out, was a kind of salamander. After an exhaustive study of its earliest stages of development, Coghill discovered that all activity of this animal originated in the musculature of its head and then flashed tailward. In other words, from the start there is a dominance of the whole over the parts. (As in Alexander, the head-neck-torso, so to speak, provides the "true and primary movement in each and every act.") Even after the animal grows and the limbs become more independent, they are still part of the "total pattern," this trunk dominance which Coghill found always to be the basic thing in the creature's movements. Coghill was certain, and there has been some later research which may tend to confirm his belief, that much the same is true of human embryonic behavior.[1] In any case, he thought that this "total pattern" in us is corrupted by the habits of civilization (and offered as a particularly striking example the custom of sitting on chairs). John Dewey commented on the magnificent bearing of men and women he had observed in South Africa and Jamaica.

The process of civilization, according to Alexander, has contaminated man's biological and sensory equipment, with a resultant crippling in the responses of the whole organism. Tension and conflict are more and more substituted for coordination. And since habits operate below the conscious level, any improvement must come through saying no to all habitual activity and supplanting it, at the physiologic level, with "the true and primary movement in each and every act." The technique which he proposed, therefore, with its kinesthetic reinstatement of a head-neck-torso coordination now lost or damaged, was directed towards what he considered the restoration of man's native condition of health.

John Dewey believed that the technique belonged to constructive education. "Its proper field of application," he wrote, "is with the young, with the growing generation, in order that they may come to possess as early as possible in life a correct standard of sensory appreciation and self-judgment." Thus they might grow up to withstand the buffetings and contingencies of civilization. Dewey's word was law to educators and teachers throughout the western world. Why then was he so disregarded on so fundamental a proposition? Aldous Huxley suggested it was because most

---

[1] The extension of Coghill's principle to human foetuses was undertaken by Davenport Hooker and Tryphena Humphrey.

educators and teachers were too kinesthetically debauched to comprehend what he was talking about.

Over and over again, in his essays and in his letters, Huxley too reverted to the educational primacy of Alexander's teaching. And in *Island,* his last novel, he sought to embody it in fictional terms. (In this final narrative, Huxley projects a bold manifesto for the future, not bothering overmuch to disguise the vision as a novel.) An interpreter from his island utopia explains to a visitor from the outside world that children may be "shown how to do things with the minimum of strain and the maximum of awareness" so that they come to enjoy even honest toil. When the visitor inquires whether all island children get this kind of training, the interpreter replies: "From the moment they start doing for themselves. For example, what's the proper way of handling yourself while you're buttoning your clothes?"

In infants, Alexander noted, before they are too extensively exposed to the influences of civilization, we may observe a superb physical functioning. The psychiatrically oriented Dr. Lawrence K. Frank, who took lessons in the technique for a year or more while serving as vice-president of the Josiah Macy Jr. Foundation, at one time tried to arrange for Alexander's brother, "A.R.," to work with a group in a New York medical school studying infant development. In his impatience with Freudian thought, John Dewey had once referred to Frank as "one of the psychologists who are led by psychoanalysts to believe that human destiny is settled in infancy by how the feeding and the excretory eliminations are treated by adults."

Dewey's apprehensions here proved unfounded. For the psychologist found Alexander's concept of inborn capacity for neuromuscular coordination not dissimilar to Freud's concept of the "primary process" which operates until learning interferes and emotional distortion overlaps its operation. The project in infant research which he conceived fell through after "A.R." demanded an exorbitant salary to participate. The unlettered Australian wanted an amount out of all proportion to what was being paid a full professor at the New York medical school involved.

Dr. Frank did, nevertheless, succeed in providing fellowships for two women to take lessons in the technique and afterwards apply this new approach to medical study. In later years, one of them produced a monograph, with fascinating photographic illustrations, which was published in *Child Study* (Vol. 9, No. 1, March 1938) under the title "A Study in Infant Development."

The interest which led her to this study, wrote Alma Frank (no relative of Dr. Frank), arose from her observation, over several years, of a gradual lessening of well-coordinated movement in young children. "At the age of two, when they entered school," she wrote, "they apparently possessed a degree of physical coordination which by the end of the third year had notably diminished; by the end of the fourth year this coordination had given way to definite well-established postural habits—rigidly fixed positions of certain parts of the body." Among the factors which reacted upon the children, Mrs. Frank included inept handling by ill-coordinated adults. And she suggested that the material she had uncovered pointed to a need for reorganizing the concepts of motor activity and the study of motor development. "The implications of this for education," she concluded, "are far-reaching."

Another of Alexander's students, Dr. Harold Schlosberg, a well-known experimental psychologist, later reiterated Mrs. Frank's insistence upon the need for sustained inquiry to settle these points. "Why do so many of us," he asked, "make this discordant tightening of the key postural muscles in the neck? Instead of sitting back in our armchairs and blaming it on vertical posture, poor training, or natural perversion, we need more research; how do the head-neck relations develop in phylogeny and in ontogeny? In other words, how do we get this way?"

In addition to the injurious effects which the normal civilizing process has upon the organism, several other explanations were brought forth by Alexander's students and associates, to account for the manner in which mankind has gone astray. Of these the most popular—to which he did not subscribe—was the now familiar hypothesis that in assuming an erect posture, the human animal, fundamentally mammalian in nature, entered upon a kind of physical crisis still unresolved. "It is highly unlikely," says Professor Tinbergen, seconding Alexander's rejection of this theory, "that in their very long evolutionary history of walking upright, the Hominids have not had time to evolve the correct mechanism for bipedal locomotion. This conclusion receives support from the surprising, but indubitable fact that even after forty to fifty years of obvious misuse, one's body can snap back into proper and in many respects more healthy use as a result of a short series of half-hourly sessions." The more drastic implications of the physical-crisis viewpoint have been definitively expressed by Theodore, the comic-grotesque, in a soliloquy entitled "Four-Leggedness—The Key to Every Lock":

*Can't you see where we are headed?*
*There is Doom in the Air and the Reek of Cooked Goose.*
*Back, back I say, back to the position Nature gave us in the Beginning.*
*Down, down I say, down on all Fours, without further ado!*
*Ado-lessly!!*

"Ado-lessly" is the exact word for what Alexander discerned as the mainspring of his technique, and he did regard it as the key to every lock, or just about every lock. But a return to primitivism of any kind was for him out of the question. No "back to Nature": no "going native." He believed that man's future was civilization. The cure for our present dilemma did not lie in any form of direct reversion to animal "instincts." It lay rather in the further extension of reason, with the paradoxical recovery—through this extension—of our vanished creature health.

This is a cardinal feature of Alexander's work which sharply differentiates it from the widespread sentimentality and anti-intellectualism of current body-practice. An essential component of his method belongs to the mind; there is a basic thinking element in it.

For to follow his method means continually saying no to all the "sets" which normally interfere with activity. It means constantly refusing all the involuntary preparations we go through which thereupon lock and impede the movements we intend. The steady process of withholding consent from these unnoticed tensions of getting ready is an inseparable part of freeing "the true and primary movement in each and every act." To a student who wrote him, "I understand I am to do nothing," Alexander replied that "to me the phrase reveals that you *do try to do nothing.*" And he pleaded with him, "Substitute for that the idea of *just refusing to do anything.*" Knowing how to stop, in short, is something that has always to be practiced and perfected in the specific situations of living. "My doing was my undoing," is how Alexander summed up his early discovery in Australia.

To the necessary denial of the unconscious panoply surrounding all that we do, Alexander applied the term "inhibition." He liked to relate how John Dewey once made a special trip to warn him against the word. It was a very bad word, Dewey told him. In the prevailing climate of psychoanalytic opinion, people were sure to confuse what he was talking about with the bad things Freud was talking about when *he* spoke of "inhibitions." Alexander would not relinquish the word, however, and in this instance at least, his choice of terminology has been vindicated by modern usage in psychology.

As he correctly recognized, the psychoanalytic use of "inhibition" has nothing to do with his meaning: within their own universe of discourse, the Freudians refer by it to the process whereby something instinctual is prevented from coming into consciousness by the activity of the superego. He on the other hand was speaking of a means for transforming the stereotyped response to a stimulus into a free choice. He meant the same thing that Sherrington did in a passage which Alexander cited to illustrate his own definition: "It has been remarked that Life's aim is an act not a thought. Today the dictum must be modified to admit that, often, to refrain from an act is no less an act than to commit one because inhibition is co-equally with excitation a nervous activity." It is not some form of going dead, or opting out: inhibition, said the neurophysiologist C. Judson Herrick, is neural vigor. In the same physiological tradition of psychology as Sherrington, a modern source-book on *Inhibition and Choice*[1] speaks of "the inhibitory mechanisms which extract unity and moderation from diversity and potential self-destructive excess."

The unspoken "orders" or "directions"[2] to which mystifying reference is occasionally made in Alexander's books were not, as might at first appear, a mode of auto-suggestion proposed to the student: they were to be silently iterated as a check on the practice of inhibition, a means for keeping track of the whole inhibitory process. Though helpful in the first stages of learning the technique, they become, in time, more and more ritualistic—a string of played-out inhibitory "Hail Mary's" gone over by rote—and tend to lose their effectiveness. Some of the newer teaching, therefore, seeks to cue the necessary inhibition not by "orders," but by any perceptual stimulus from one's surroundings—a sound, a color, a sensation. It may be the whir of an electric fan, the tint of a curtain, a feeling of heaviness in one's elbows from leaning upon them, anything at all which happens to register clearly.

To inhibit implies an awareness of the bodily "sets" to be inhibited. Awareness and the power to inhibit increase side by side, reinforcing one another, and together allowing the "primary movement" to operate. The freefloating effect of the technique comes about only as the result of these. However tempting to try to do so, one cannot either hang onto or seize that effect by itself. "Throw it away!" Alexander always exclaimed the moment a student began to exult over his sense of weightlessness. "One of my greatest handicaps," wrote Dewey in a letter, "was that after I got the lightness sensory effect I would try to keep *it* instead of the means-whereby." We should learn to think, he said, always in terms of the present participle, not in the past-participle: go on with the continuing activity of "standing," for example, not stay put in a condition of "having stood." Every fresh sensation of lightness, therefore, has a newly minted quality, unpredictable, here-now, unique, and occurs outside of and beyond any direct striving for it. A feasible new name has been suggested as a replacement for the vague old name of "Alexander technique." There seems no reason why the method may not be known as "AGR facilitation," if it be understood that in this facilitation of the anti-gravity response is included the inhibitory coopera-tion of the student.

---

[1] Diamond, S., Balvin, R. S., & Diamond, F.R.
[2] For one version of these "orders," see page xxiii above.

As Alexander rightly insisted, then, inhibition was the very word he needed to designate the process which releases—rather than imprisons—spontaneity. It is the process which intensifies, rather than diminishes, our satisfaction in activity. It "increases rather than reduces gratification."

Alexander rejected the possibility of putting salt on the bird's tail: this bird eludes straight capture. Not through the directness of excitation but through the indirectness of inhibition is it to be caught. As many present-day followers of "sensory awakening" and "touch therapy" have begun to discover, there are few things more rigid than programmatic spontaneity. The Alexander technique is "consciousness expanding" all right, but it is at the same time a discipline: it makes one more aware of inner powers, but at the same time provides a means for realizing them. "Thinking in activity" was thus another name by which Alexander, following Dewey, sometimes called "the work." It was setting your knowledge in motion. And after his development of a means for conveying kinesthetic experience, this discovery about the role of inhibition in the integration of reflex and voluntary movement ranks as the next most important part of his work.

To make it easy to talk about the whole process, Alexander came up with two new terms, highly focused and greatly helpful (when applied to the exact specifics of "the work," and not used as abstract philosophic generalities to rationalize the major and minor decisions of human existence). "Endgaining" is the immediate response which follows upon the innervation of the muscles which habitually perform an act. Attention to the "means-whereby" refers to the instant of pause or refusal or inhibition which disallows that immediate response. In these simple terms, Alexander was able to bring home his message: forgetting about the endgain, while concentrating our all on the means-whereby.

"What he means is not forgetting," wrote Dr. Frederick Perls from South Africa in 1944, "but a temporary pushing aside of the endgain." Using Alexander's favorite example of golf, he pointed out that the golfer who forgets the *aim* of his endeavors, concentrating only on the means-whereby—how to hold on to the club, how to turn his wrist—will lose interest and stop playing golf altogether. Or else he may become involved in meaningless dummy-activity. So too, continued Perls, it is of course true, as Alexander maintains, that you will not become a musician merely by striving for the endgain: to be a great artist. At best you will become a talented amateur. But it is equally true that if you concentrate purely on the means-whereby, which is to say on technique—and you forget entirely about the endgain, which is to say, the appreciation, reproduction and perhaps composition, of music—your practicing will become mechanical and meaningless. At best you may become a virtuoso.

During actual lessons in "the work," this question about totally forgetting the endgain does not perhaps matter so much. The teacher knows the endgain and will see to it, no matter how exclusively the student may be concentrating on the means-whereby, that he does stand up or sit down or walk or climb stairs or perform whatever other act may be required of him. With his hands, the teacher feels what is happening, detects if the "sets" are being sensed and inhibited, and initiates the proper directions for the movements to take place, at the same time indicating if necessary that some wrong action is under way.

But when you are on your own, Dr. Perls explained, it is important to keep the interdependency of aim and technique in mind. "You have," he said, "to find out 'how' you react in detail (the structure of the means-whereby); to realize these details you must feel them (the sensory appreciation). If during the process you 'forget' the endgain, you will condition yourself to a flight of ideas. Such forgetting of aims (aimless talking or doing) is a symptom of insanity. You will appreciate that the difference between 'forgetting the endgain' and 'keeping it in the background' is not a quibbling over words, but entails a decisive difference of meaning."

Perls, afterwards to be known as the father of Gestalt therapy, was then a Captain in the wartime South African Medical Corps. He was the founder of the South African Institute for Psychoanalysis in Johannesburg, and his deeply appreciative critique of Alexander, contained in a book titled *Ego, Hunger and Aggression,* published in Durban, provides some measure of the strong influence the technique was having in South African medical and scientific circles.

Socially, Alexander believed that the human organism has many potentials which may be developed for good or ill. His proposal for the proper use of the self through recovery of its "true and primary movement" he offered as a means to activate these potentials in a desirable way. It was a way which led to making a person self-consciously aware of, and thereby liberated from, unconscious processes. His technique provided a means of escape from the chains of habit. Free of habit, people would be capable of choice. They could act with responsibility for his actions.

Alexander viewed the technique not merely as a hopeful prospect for the individual, however. Even into the age of the atom bomb, which he lived to see, he continued to locate and preach the salvation of humankind in such a development. (He was an unrelenting Germanophobe, and there was always some question whether the Germans might not have to be left behind unsaved.) The adoption of conscious guidance and control as a universal principle, he declared, "will enable us to move slowly but with gradually increasing speed towards those higher psychophysical spheres which will separate the animal and human kingdoms by a deep gulf, and mankind will then enjoy the blessings which will be the natural result of capacities fully developed." John Dewey, who saw in education the only sure method which mankind possesses for directing its own course, in effect agreed. For he held that the technique bears the same relationship to education as education itself bears to other activities.

Can there be anyone left today who does not concede the truth in Randolph Bourne's early assessment (see p. xviii) of this scheme for saving the world (an assessment which applies with later and greater force, however, to the many other psychophysical schemes for saving the world now current and being promulgated, some of them, under fairly prestigious auspices)? "For if this next step in evolution is to mean anything," said Bourne, "it means that every separate human being must make over his bodily coordinations." And if we must all await the consummation of this appalling social task—if we must wait till everyone has learned conscious guidance and control—then indeed, as Bourne remarked with gentle irony, "the next step in evolution will be very long delayed."

To expect in fact that any changes whatever in the techniques and methods of educators, rather than in the society which supports them, will now transform the world is no longer a serious viewpoint. The impact of events has proved Alexander, and Dewey as well, hopelessly wrong about that—woefully, grievously wrong. Not even a writer like Arthur Koestler, who along with Alexander attributed the world crisis to an evolutionary gap, placed his hope in any type of educational reform but rather (an opposite wistful extreme) in the future discovery and rapid popularization of some drug which will remedy the gap.

All the same, Alexander's transcendent faith in the redemptive power of reason upon history was an astonishing end point to be reached by a man who was himself a species of "primitive." This after all was the kind of man who could assert without the least trace of embarrassment: "I don't care what man you bring up, Socrates or anyone else, you will find gaps and holes in his thinking. Let me coordinate him and you will not find gaps and holes in his thinking." He was a figure comparable to the self-taught painter in art. He was the typical hermit-discoverer: the man who has found out something all by himself without benefit of laboratory or research set-up. If his teaching now seems more acceptable—or at any rate less bizarre—than it once did, that is only because he was followed by a long line of thinkers who have more "respectably" familiarized us with the kind of thing he was talking about: Hans Selye with his concept of stress, and the general adaptation syndrome, whereby the defenses and resources of the total organism are mobilized to resist infection and traumas; Paul Schilder with his concept of "body image," and the three-dimensional picture we have of ourselves; Wilhelm Reich with his concept of "bodily armoring," the muscular inflexibility with which we defend ourselves against a world which seems threatening.

The school of psychosomatic medicine, in fact, grew up only during his lifetime. And the various schools in psychiatry which approach the psyche by way of the body have only recently come into full swing. We are no longer so quizzical about an external approach, like Alexander's, to worry, anxiety, fear and other states of emotion. "All of the 'psychic' complexes have their basis in organic discoordinations and tensions, with compensatory flabbinesses," Dewey wrote in an early letter, "and his technique is a technique for resolving and unraveling those, reducing the present technique of the psychoanalyst to an incidental accompaniment, and cutting out the elaborate ritualistic mummery with which the present psychoanalysts have been obliged to surround their method. In addition, Mr. Alexander's technique unravels the kinks and complexes by a process of positive replacement in which sound coordinations are built up with their corresponding alterations in habitual sensory and emotional data, while at the best the psychoanalysts merely untie a knot and leave the organic causes which produced it untouched."

Aldous Huxley was in solid agreement. He pointed out that many undesirable mental states may be traced, not to some traumatic event of childhood or the more recent past, but to what Alexander called "the improper use of the self," resulting in impaired physiological and psychological functioning. "If you teach an individual," wrote Huxley, "first to be aware of his physical organism and then to use it as it was meant to be used, you can often change his entire attitude to life and cure his neurotic tendencies. But this, of course, is something which no one-sided psychologist has been taught to do, or would approve of doing, even if he knew how. He just goes on with free association and dream analysis, and hopes for the best. And the best (as those who have tried to assess the effectiveness of psychoanalysis assure us) does not happen as often as one might hope or, given the exorbitant cost of the treatment, legitimately expect."

Lewis Mumford set Alexander's work within the context that self-knowledge may be approached from either the outside or the inside, by way of the body or by way of the mind. Provided that one pushes far enough, he explained, one will find the unrepresented portions reappearing in the full description. "Alexander's approach to the self," wrote Mumford, "begins with the human body as the outward manifestation of every inward tendency... Since we have abundant evidence to show that in many cases psychological interpretation has removed physical symptoms there is no reason to doubt that the reverse method of approach, correcting the psyche by means of studied bodily readjustments, may be equally effective."

During his lifetime, in fact, Alexander became acquainted with, and ardently applauded, what William James then was saying about "ideo-motor function"—that is, the dynamics of conscious attitude and image in giving shape and direction to posture, and movement to the muscles of the body. As early as 1908, eight years before Alexander's first meeting with Dewey, he was using James's concept and term in his writing. An anticipated encounter with James never materialized because of the latter's death in 1910. (He did make the acquaintance of the novelist-brother, Henry James.)

The psychiatrist Frederick Perls held that Alexander and Freud had independently discovered the need for detailed analysis and complete consciousness of those rooted subdivisions of the human personality which we take for granted and justify as "force of habit," "character," "constitution" and the like. But these characteristics have a very stubborn, conservative tendency, he noted; and he gave full credit to Alexander for recognizing, along with Freud, that they do not change of their own accord, that they cannot be reorganized without conscious concentration. "Without this reorganization," said Perls, "no reconstruction of the personality can be achieved."

Yet Alexander remained a primitive. He was always the man who just *knew*. "Stupid!" was a favorite epithet of his for everyone and everything, and too often "Stupid" came to signify his exasperation with the pedestrian steps of verification needed in science. He was capable of downright silliness about it: he could say that he had been discouraged from seeking a physiological explanation of his work when he observed the manner in which some physiologists carried themselves. Though his work evoked words of praise from titans of scientific thought like Sherrington and Coghill, though the Chairman of the Representative Body of the British Medical Association staunchly supported him, though at one point the *British Medical Journal* even published a letter signed by nineteen physicians calling upon their profession to recognize and evaluate the technique because of its remarkable effectiveness in treating many of their patients—through it all and to the end, he remained suspicious of the prevailing scientific approach. Perhaps with some justice, he viewed the science of his day as too analytical, fracturing the whole man into parts and then studying the relations of the variables. No amount of such analysis, he was convinced, could yield any real understanding of the human organism and its capacity for integrated functioning in the environment.

Apart from such legitimate differences in principle, however, it is also true that he effectually repulsed much of the important financial and technical help that was offered him. Dewey, after trying repeatedly to bring him into fruitful connection with the world of foundations and university research, finally gave up. Dewey never wavered in his judgment of the technique's validity ("having living proof in myself") but in the end decided that real investigation of it could never proceed during the inventor's lifetime. Another student, Sir Stafford Cripps, likewise abandoned the effort to establish a well-organized teaching center with Alexander's cooperation: Cripps made the attempt alone. Alexander turned thumbs down hard on the inception of a research project at Harvard Medical School. The prospect of entrusting investigation to researchers even of the magnitude of the child specialist Arnold Gesell did not impress him. For he distrusted not science but scientists. He knew what he had: but he knew not what it might become at their hands. He likewise sabotaged a research grant from the Rockefeller Foundation which influential friends sought for "the work."

In the way of a poor man who had worked hard and long to secure a good livelihood (for himself and others), he took an objective view of how monies are divided up and apportioned in the "projects" conducted by universities and foundations. To them his discovery might provide an endlessly significant topic for research. But it was his bread and butter (or lobster and wine), and he never for one moment lost sight of that brutal material fact.

His grandiloquent personal style—for there was a bit of the ham as well as of the actor in him—with its sweeping claims of prodigious cures and amazing transformations, also helped to estrange a number of his more conservative colleagues who were otherwise sympathetic to his approach. He did not hesitate to pronounce ex-cathedra judgments on such portentous matters as cancer and the dismal future of cancer research.

Yet despite all this, it would be a cardinal error to think that Alexander looked anywhere else for approval than to the rationalist scientific tradition in which he was rooted. Born a decade after publication of *The Origin of Species*, he had begun as a Darwinian, and as a follower of Herbert Spencer and T.H. Huxley, at a time when it took courage for an unschooled young Australian to hold such views. He wholeheartedly seized upon the researches of the physiologist Rudolph Magnus, dealing with the "attitudinal" and "righting" reflexes in animals. (It was from a misinterpretation of something in Magnus that he coined the unfortunate phrase "primary control" to designate what he had previously called "the true and primary movement."[1]) He diligently sought to have an understanding of his technique included in the orthodox medical practice of his time. If only they would see that the condition of the whole self is a limiting factor on any activity! If only they would see that if you are going to treat symptoms, you must be thoroughly aware of their integration, actual or potential, with the whole system! That orthodox practice he accepted, when needed, for himself and his family. He did not, for example, follow Aldous Huxley into the supernal reaches of the healing arts and remonstrated with him, earnestly and at length, in opposition to such things as his espousal of the Bates method for improving eyesight. (It is true that J.E.R. McDonagh, whose medical credentials were conventional but whose methods were not, he valued as a colleague—but Alexander himself was too much the gourmet to abide McDonagh's special diet.)

The monumental self-assurance, the stolid pride, the curious dignity of the man, which throughout his lifetime precluded the slightest innuendo of charlatanism or quackery in his presence, were founded upon a rational certainty of where he stood. It was with absolute confidence that, in late years, he launched upon the suit for defamation against his public detractor in South Africa—a German, the man was, besides!—and throughout the immense, complicated and interminable litigation which followed, he arduously pursued his course without any real doubt as to the eventual outcome: the decision in his own favor. For him the issue was never in question.

Students of Alexander's like the Archbishop of Canterbury, William Temple, might equate his technique with the Divine Creativity of Christian faith (as students would one day, after his death, discern in its lighter-than-air "ado-less" dynamism the *satori* of Zen). He was tolerant of that kind of thing, even sympathetic towards it, and of course he always welcomed favor or attention from whatever source. "If there is a crackpot within fifty miles," he once told a teacher, "he will find his way to me." But all that stood clearly outside his own rationalist perspective.

He looked indifferently away from any religious, occult, mystagogical or esoteric sanction of his work. Yoga, meditation, hypnosis, auto-suggestion and the like were, all of them, anathema to him. Such practices he regarded as catering to levels of the unconscious, a species of "demoralization." His

---

[1] Magnus emphasized that no direct control is possible. Alexander's is, rather, a method of indirect control, a means of facilitating the "primary movement," which is to say the action of these reflexes. See Appendix III, pages 197–200.

absolute detestation of Gerald Heard as a purveyor of these enormities (apart from the fact that Heard did not come to him as a student) sprang from his stern rationalist bias.

"You see," he explained to one correspondent, "a person cannot capitulate to subconscious guidance to the extent which 'meditation' demands in practice, without seriously affecting the psychophysical self in reaction to living." It is a supreme irony that the fictional portrait of Alexander which has come down to us—in Huxley's *Eyeless in Gaza*—should be an amalgam of Alexander and Gerald Heard (who also provided an impetus, though one of a decidedly different kind, to the novelist's life). Most literary studies today—for example, Professor George Woodcock's book on Huxley, where Alexander is presented as the guru who "introduced him to effective techniques of meditation"—continue to perpetuate the outlandish confusion of these two opposite figures. In a book of popular mysticism, Alan Watts places the technique in a heterogeneous catalog which includes yoga meditation, dervish dancing, Zen Buddhism, Ignatian, Salesian and Hesychest methods of "prayer," the use of consciousness-changing chemicals such as LSD and mescalin, Quakerism, Gurdjieff exercises and self-hypnosis. Heard, it is true, did have kind words to say about Alexander somewhere in his writing, but there was not the slightest degree of consanguinity felt on the other side. Bernard Shaw, no great mystic himself, concurred with his teacher in a gruff discussion they held about the man.

Now that the technique has begun to take popular hold, a fresh variety of views is being brought to bear upon it. At Tufts University, Professor Frank Pierce Jones and his associates, using a battery of sophisticated equipment, for many years conducted research designed to cast light on the underlying principles of the method. By means of stroboscopic photography and electromyography, they were able to demonstrate the specific alteration in movement patterns that can be produced by the technique. Sheaves and sheaves of impressive before-and-after posture photos can be had from almost every known school of exercise or relaxation today (pictures which remain quite without serious evidential value). Unlike such posture stills, the methods evolved by the Tufts group were designed to register a precise index of change; and they showed that the technique obtains results—within movement—which may not be duplicable by any non-Alexandrian type of reeducation, and which cannot be faked.

Jones believed that too much attention has been paid to Alexander's technique and philosophy and too little to his discovery. In his view, Alexander discovered a mechanism for achieving a higher integration of human responses—namely, that in the presence of a stimulus to move, the inhibition of certain postural sets facilitates the anti-gravity reflexes. This principle he sought to formulate in terms which would bring it into the domain of empirical investigation and continuing research.

Jones's last projects involved the use of sound spectrograms ("voice-prints") to demonstrate the effect of the technique on vocal resonance and breath control, and of a strain-gauge force platform to measure the way force is applied in initiating movement. If one stands with one foot on the force platform and the other on a dummy platform beside it, it will measure the preliminary shift in weight—that is, the "set"—when one steps off it. From sitting to standing, it measures the difference in the amount of force used in a technique-guided as opposed to a habitual movement. Jones also developed a comprehensive and intelligible theory of the head-neck-torso pattern in terms of known and studied postural reflexes.[1] Presently needed is a sound, careful and thorough scientific evaluation of Jones's work. Computerized movement analysis will now simplify future research.

So Alexander stands today: a stubborn genius who uncovered a valuable mechanism for human growth; who then evolved an imperfect technique for imparting the experience of that mechanism to others; and who from the mechanism and the technique, so full of promise for both the physical and emotional development of the individual, inferred a fanciful program of evolutionary repair which in the present critical world state scarcely warrants respectful attention. The challenge of developing more and more effective versions of the technique remains with us, however, for future fulfillment. "I wish to do away with such teachers as I am myself," the inventor himself once wrote.

For the abrupt reemergence today of this lively, obscured heritage from Alexander, there may be urgent cause. In the most premonitory myth of modern times, the science of Frankenstein spawns a monster human: not the ghoul we think, but the first innocent child of machine technology. Science's most recent child is the younger, more helpless generation of the electronic era, when the very physical-being of the person, fast on its way to replacement, is called into question.

"A strange multiplicity of sensations seized me," explains the monster in Mary Shelley's touching novella, recalling the tremulous days before he turned against the whole world in a rage of destruction, "and I saw, felt, heard and smelt at the same time.... Sometimes I wished to express my sensations in my own mode, but the uncouth and inarticulate sounds which broke from me frightened me into silence again."

[1] Appendix III.

Here now comes Alexander again, with that curious idea of his for instructing Frankenstein's baby in the flesh-and-blood fundamentals of its new condition. Who knows? For many today, living in cities, working indoors mostly at sedentary, small-muscle jobs, continually exposed to polluted air, and hampered in opportunities for any large recreation—for many of this latest brood of monsters, it could just turn the trick.

EDWARD MAISEL

# BIBLIOGRAPHIC NOTE

The selections which follow have, with one exception, been taken from the four books which Alexander wrote: *Man's Supreme Inheritance* (1910); *Constructive Conscious Control of the Individual* (1923); *The Use of the Self* (1932); and *The Universal Constant in Living* (1941).

Prior to 1910, Alexander had published three short essays on his work in the form of pamphlets. In 1912, he published a short book called *Conscious Control*, which in 1918 was incorporated in a new edition of *Man's Supreme Inheritance*. The manuscript of *Constructive Conscious Control of the Individual*, which Alexander regarded as his best book, was carefully gone over by John Dewey and Dr. Peter Macdonald. *The Use of the Self* also went through Dewey's hands in manuscript form.

Alexander wrote most of *The Universal Constant in Living,* his last book, before departure for America in 1940. He then finished the book during a three-month holiday at Southwest Harbour, Maine, where he stayed with friends. Coghill, who wrote the introduction, was living in retirement at Gainesville, Florida, where in 1941 he met Alexander.

The selection included here under the title "After the Bomb" appeared originally in the revised edition of *The Universal Constant in Living* which was published in 1946, and served as Alexander's foreword to a symposium on his work published the same year. The crisp and lively "Notes of Instruction," which contain the epitome of the technique, have been chosen from a longer transcript made during Alexander's actual teaching sessions with a variety of students. These are published here for the first time.

Some of the selections presented have been woven from strands extracted from the four books and combined and edited so as to bear upon a single topic. Minor changes such as a shift in the tense of a verb, the omission of a transitional phrase, the carrying over of a clause from one paragraph to the next, the breaking up of a sentence, and similar devices have been resorted to where necessary in order to accomplish this unity of design. Nevertheless care has been taken not to tamper with the author's personal style. The original orthography (for example, "shew" for "show") has likewise been retained throughout. Only new chapter titles have been provided to conform with the new arrangement of material.

Frank Pierce Jones's formal explanation of the Alexander technique and his researches into it (Appendix III, pp. xliii–xliv) are still the best we have. Despite the warm endorsement by Professor Niko Tinbergen in his 1973 Nobel address, it promulgated a cardinal misconception of the technique as "no more than...corrective manipulation of the entire muscular system" and "a mere gentle handling of the body muscles." Tinbergen offered moving testimony to what the technique had done for him and his family; he made astute comments on Alexander's mode of discovery, and offered before-and-after photographs of Alexander technique students. Yet Alexander himself was against such photographic evidence. On October 27, 1952, he wrote disapprovingly about Dr. Wilfred Barlow (a follower with whom he broke during his last years): "I have intimated my objection to his 'conditioning' and photographs as means of proof." Barlow's attempts to associate the technique with Pavlovian conditioning have long since been forgotten. But scientifically naive before-and-after photographs persist; indeed, it was Barlow's photographs which Tinbergen displayed in his Nobel presentation.[1]

[1] Readers interested in the technicalities of the Nobel episode are referred to my critique of Tinbergen (*Science:* Vol. 188, No. 4187, pp. 404–5, Vol. 188, No. 4192, p. 974) and to the extended discussion in *New Scientist,* involving Tinbergen, New Scientist editor Dr. Roger Lewin, Patrick J. Macdonald, Barlow, myself and others (*New Scientist:* Vol. 64, No. 921, p. 344; Vol. 64, No. 923, p. 524; Vol. 64, No. 925, pp. 679–80; Vol. 64, No. 926, pp. 772–3; Vol. 64, No. 927, p. 839; Vol. 64, No. 928, p. 895; Vol. 65, No. 932, p. 160).

# ACKNOWLEDGMENTS

There is no reliable biography of Alexander, nor is there any definitive book about his work. During the twelve years in which I have been looking into these subjects, I have had to rely upon a voluminous quantity of original material.

For their cooperation and generosity in making available letters, diaries, reminiscences and other first-hand data, I should like to thank here a number of persons who helped me: Mrs. Arthur J. Busch, Mrs. John Dewey, Robert van Geuns, Walter H.M. Carrington, Patrick J. Macdonald, Dr. Wilfred Barlow, Judith Leibowitz, Goddard Binkley, Joan Murray, Deborah Caplan, Richard M. Gummere, Jr., Eric de Peyer, Margaret Goldie, Irene Tasker, Edward Owen, Marjorie Barstow, Michael Frederick, Peter Trimmer, and Dr. Richard A. Brown.

I should also like to record the assistance of three persons who have died since this book was started: Father Eric D. McCormack, Lulie Westfeldt, and with utmost gratitude for his incredibly extended advice and patience in piecing together bits of the missing record, Dr. Lawrence K. Frank.

Apart from extremely useful discussion, Professor Otto Jokl made available to me complete transcripts of the South African court proceedings.

Beaumont Alexander and J.A. Alexander offered the necessary permission for reproduction of the selections I have chosen to offer here.

At the Institute for Psychological Research at Tufts University, Professor Frank Pierce Jones and his associates were most gracious in acquainting me with the experimental work which was conducted there during a good quarter of a century. The Wessell Library at Tufts University did everything possible to expedite my handling of the Dewey correspondence on Alexander which is lodged there. The *Psychological Review* kindly granted permission to offer as an appendix my own abridgment of a paper by Professor Jones which first appeared in their pages (Vol. 72, No. 3, May 1965).

Having expressed this considerable indebtedness, I hasten to add that I alone bear full responsibility for all statements and viewpoints embodied in the present work.

E.M.

. . . my experience may one day be recognized as a signpost directing the explorer to a country hitherto "undiscovered," and one which offers unlimited opportunity for fruitful research to the patient and observant pioneer.

F. Matthias Alexander

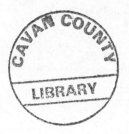

# PART I
# THE TECHNIQUE

## Chapter One

# NOTES OF INSTRUCTION

*(addressed to a variety of students during actual teaching sessions)*

This isn't breathing; it's lifting your chest and collapsing.

---

I see at last that if I don't breathe, I breathe . . .

---

If I breathe as I understand breathing, I am doing something wrong.

---

Control should be in process, not superimposed.

---

You ask me to lift that chair. If I give consent that is all I can do.

---

You can't change the course of nature by co-ordinating yourself.

---

You've been trying to use your organism by primarily dis-coordinating it.

---

They may have an intellectual conception of what they want, and they may write down what they want to bring about, but how are they going to do it? They are not doing *the* thing that alters the rest.

---

Change involves carrying out an activity against the habit of life.

---

Take hold of the floor with your feet. What can that mean to them? When they try to take hold of the floor with their feet, they take half the foot off the floor with the tension they are putting on their legs.

---

When you are asked not to do something, instead of making

the decision not to do it, you try to prevent yourself from doing it. But this only means that you decide to do it, and then use muscle tension to prevent yourself from doing it.

---

The things that don't exist are the most difficult to get rid of.

---

It's not getting in and out of chairs even under the best of conditions that is of any value; that is simply physical culture—it is what you have been doing in preparation that counts when it comes to making movements.

---

There is no such thing as a right position, but there is such a thing as a right direction.

---

Everything a person has done in the past has been in accordance with the mental direction to which he is accustomed, and it is his faith in this that makes him unwilling to exchange it for the new direction one is trying to give him.

---

You can speak as well as I can, except that you are doing something to speak that no one does except people who stammer like you.

---

You are doing what you call "leaving yourself alone."

---

Doing in your case is so "overdoing" that you are practically paralysing the parts you want to work.

---

You want to think the devil of a time before you do it because the old idea of doing comes back to us.

---

You can't tell a person what to do, because the thing you have to do is a sensation.

---

What you feel is doing is "undoing."

---

These things can take care of themselves.

---

All the damned fools in the world believe they are actually doing what they think they are doing.

———

You can't do something you don't know, if you keep on doing what you do know.

———

You are not making decisions: you are doing kinesthetically what you feel to be right.

———

I ask you to do nothing, but you act as if I had asked you to do. I have got to train you to act according to your decision where the habits of life are concerned.

———

The important thing is what the child is doing with itself in its activities.

———

Everyone is always teaching one what to do, leaving us still doing the things we shouldn't do.

———

The experience you want is in the process of getting it. If you have something, give it up. Getting it, not having it, is what you want.

———

Under the ordinary teaching methods, the pupil gets nineteen wrong and one right experience. It ought to be the other way round.

———

Mr. S. came in and said he had trouble with his eyes. He spent three days in bed, when he found his eyes working quite normally, and this continued all the time he was in bed. As soon as he got up again and began walking about, his eyes went wrong again.

———

You say it is wrong for the boy to be frightened. I say you are wrong in saying so. I should say it would be serious if he were not frightened when he is in the condition he is.

———

Any fool can do the thing he wants to feel—there is no trouble about that. The difficulty is to make him feel he does not want to feel.

---

If your neck feels stiff, that is not to say your neck "is" stiff.

---

I should make mistakes if I reacted to some new things as you do . . . the thing we are trying to kill in you is your "individuality," and we can't do it. Individuality is a habit.

---

You get away from your old preconceived ideas because you are getting away from your old habits.

---

We can throw away the habit of a lifetime in a few minutes if we use our brains.

---

They won't try and get out of the chair unless they feel they have that something that will get them out of the chair: that something is their habit.

---

When I ask you to draw your tongue away and say "t", I mean you not to say "t". I mean you definitely to prevent it, to give orders, and not to say "t". I ask you to say "t" because I don't want you to say "t", because I want to give you the opportunity of refusing to say "t".

---

Prevent the things you have been doing and you are half way home.

---

You are doing something you are not asked to do. Don't you see that what you call the impossibility never arises unless you do the thing you are not supposed to do.

---

They say, "I am going to lengthen," and then raise their eyes. Of course raising their eyes has nothing more to do with lengthening than their boots, but having done this from time onwards, their conception of lengthening will be associated with raising their eyes. Therefore when the idea of lengthening comes to them, they must at once inhibit the movement of the eyes in order to break the wrong association that has been built up, before giving themselves the order to lengthen.

———————

You can't know a thing by an instrument that's wrong.

———————

As soon as people come with the ideas of unlearning instead of learning, you have them in the frame of mind you want.

———————

If people will go on believing that they "know", it is impossible to eradicate anything: it makes it impossible to teach them.

———————

Link up your message and the feeling of it now. When you have learnt that, you have learnt the thing by means of which you do any exercise.

———————

The point is that "intellectuality" as we understand it, means it can only be used when we are wrong within us.

———————

It's there in all the other thinking. When you get in a dilemma, you don't lose it. It means that the thing that helps you in a crisis becomes "conscious".

———————

I am putting into gear the muscles that hold up, and you are putting them out of gear and then making a tremendous effort to hold yourself up, with the result that, when you cease that effort, you slump down worse than ever.

———————

When an investigation comes to be made, it will be found that every single thing we are doing in the work is exactly what is being done in Nature where the conditions are right, the difference being that we are learning to do it consciously.

———————

He gets what he feels is the right position, but that only means that he's getting the position which fits in with his defective co-ordination.

———————

We are forced in our teaching at every point to translate theories into concrete processes.

———————

The person who prays to have help in getting rid of something will never make the effort to get rid of it.

---

If you apply the principle to the carrying out of one evolution, you have learned the lot.

---

The difficulty for all of us is to take up a new way of life in which we must apply principles instead of the haphazard end-gaining methods of the past. This indicates a slow process and we must all be content with steady improvement from day to day; but we must see to it that we are really depending upon the application of our principles in all our endeavours in every direction from day to day. You have been too anxious to be right despite the fact that you learned early in your lessons that your right was wrong. However you have done well considering your difficulties, and you will continue to improve in the controlled use of yourself if you work as steadily as directed.

---

They prevent the very ideals in which they say they believe from materializing, by the principles on which they work.

---

The essence of the religious outlook is that religion should not be kept in a compartment by itself, but that it should be the ever-present guiding principle underlying the "daily round", the "common task". So also it is possible to apply this principle of life in the daily round of one's activities without involving a loss of attention in these activities.

---

I can do the best I can for you, and if you don't know it and don't understand it, you will react to me as if I were your enemy.

---

Suppose you had the power to change a thief by magic, it would be of no use. The man would have had no experience in resisting temptation (that is, no experience of reacting rightly or wrongly to certain stimuli, and reacting ninety-nine times rightly to once wrongly), which is the experience a man must get before he can change from being a thief.

---

No one could be satisfied to go on every day getting no result unless he saw the way.

---

If you do anything to affect the processes, you must do something that will affect the results of these processes.

---

You all believe that you must know whether you are right or wrong if you are to make progress.

---

You are not here to do exercises, or to learn to do something right, but to get able to meet a stimulus that always puts you wrong and to learn to deal with it.

---

You come to learn to inhibit and to direct your activity. You learn, first, to inhibit the habitual reaction to certain classes of stimuli, and second, to direct yourself consciously in such a way as to affect certain muscular pulls, which processes bring about a new reaction to these stimuli. Boiled down, it all comes to inhibiting a particular reaction to a given stimulus. But no one will see it that way. They will all see it as getting in and out of a chair the right way. It is nothing of the kind. It is that a pupil decides what he will or will not consent to do. They may teach you anatomy and physiology till they are black in the face—you will still have this to face, sticking to a decision against your habit of life.

---

The right thing to do would be the last thing we should do, left to ourselves, because it would be the last thing we should think it would be the right thing to do.

---

You all want to know if you're right. When you get further on you will be right, but you won't know it and won't want to know if you're right.

---

You want to feel out whether you are right or not. I am giving you a conception to eradicate that. I don't want you to care a damn if you're right or not. Directly you don't care if you're right or not, the impeding obstacle is gone.

---

The old idea of trying to be right has remained with us, in spite of the fact that conditions have changed and our right is wrong.

---

The stupidity of letting children go wrong is that once they go wrong, their right is wrong; therefore the more they try to be right, the more they go wrong.

---

Don't come to me unless, when I tell you you are wrong, you make up your mind to smile and be pleased.

---

When people are wrong, the thing that is right is bound to be wrong to them.

---

Here you are, a young fellow of seventeen, knowing that you are wrong, as I know you are. Doesn't that show that your "right" is wrong, for you never tried to be wrong? You were always trying to be right. All I want you to do is to give certain directions for me, and then inhibit the tremendous effort you are making to be right.

---

To know when we are wrong is all that we shall ever know in this world.

---

Don't you see that if you "get" perfection today, you will be farther away from perfection than you have ever been?

---

Directly you get to the point where they are right, they won't go on—there is no urge—they don't want to go on. That means that all energy and accomplishment can only be used when it is accompanied by the wrong thing.

---

When anything is pointed out, our only idea is to go from wrong to right in spite of the fact that it has taken us years to get wrong: we try to get right in a moment.

---

Like a good fellow, stop the things that are wrong first.

---

The minute you change it, the thing that isn't a strain feels a strain.

---

Everyone wants to be right, but no one stops to consider if their idea of right is right.

---

There is so much to be seen when one reaches the point of being able to see, and the experience makes the meat it feeds on.

---

People that haven't any fish to fry, they see it all right.

---

When people are wrong, the thing which is right is bound to be wrong to them.

---

All that I am trying to give you is a new experience.

---

He gets what he feels is the right position, but when he has an imperfect co-ordination he is only getting a position which fits with his defective co-ordination.

---

You won't energize to put your head forward and up, unless you feel the condition which you associate with the idea of head forward and up, which is, unfortunately, stiffening and shortening, the very opposite of forward and up.

---

He is getting to the stage when things are happening. He was at the stage before when things were beginning to happen, and he was enjoying feeling them. Now he has got past that and he thinks that nothing is happening.

---

Sensory appreciation conditions conception—you can't know a thing by an instrument that is wrong.

---

When the time comes that you can trust your feeling, you won't want to use it.

---

It doesn't alter a fact because you can't feel it.

---

Be careful of the printed matter: you may not read it as it is written down.

---

As a matter of fact, feeling is much more use than what they call "mind" when it's right.

———————

If I went to a man to take singing lessons, it wouldn't matter what he taught me, he couldn't injure me.

———————

What you gain in one way you lose in another. Therefore you must not try for specific results.

———————

Specific prevention is permissible only under conditions of non-doing, not in doing.

———————

The whole organism is responsible for specific trouble. Proof of this is, that we eradicate specific defects in process.

———————

You translate everything, whether physical or mental or spiritual, into muscular tension.

———————

Trying is only emphasizing the thing we know already.

———————

Talk about a man's individuality and character: it's the way he uses himself.

———————

*Chapter Two*

# BASIC PROCEDURE

The problem before us is to find a *means whereby* a reliable sensory appreciation can be developed and maintained throughout the organism, and the basis for my argument is that both in education and in re-education this must be brought about in every case by the reliance of the individual, not upon subconscious, but upon *conscious, reasoning* guidance and control.

For we find that the human creature, subjected to the present processes of civilization, develops defects and imperfections in the use of the organism, even in cases where a reliable sensory appreciation *has already existed* on a subconscious basis, whilst in the much larger number of cases, where defects have already been developed, we find that satisfactory results cannot be secured unless during the process a new and reliable sensory appreciation is being gradually acquired. Almost all civilized human creatures have developed a condition in which the sensory appreciation (feeling) is more or less imperfect and deceptive, and it naturally follows that it cannot be relied upon in re-education, readjustment and co-ordination, or in our attempts to put right something we know to be wrong with our psycho-physical selves. The connexion[1] between psycho-physical defects and incorrect sensory guidance must therefore be recognized by the teacher in the practical work of re-education. This recognition will make it impossible for him to expect a pupil to be able to perform satisfactorily any new psycho-physical act *until the new correct experiences in sensory appreciation involved have become established.*

I will now endeavour to outline as clearly as possible the general scheme which I advocate in connexion with the development of reliable sensory appreciation. First, this scheme demands in particular on the part of the teacher a recognition of the almost alarming dominance of the pupil's psycho-physical processes by an incorrect sensory appreciation during the attempted performance

[1] The recognition of this vital connexion marks the point of departure between methods of teaching on a conscious and on a subconscious basis.

of any psycho-physical activity. It is therefore of primary importance that the teacher should recognize and endeavour to awaken his pupil to the fact of his (the pupil's) unreliable sensory appreciation, and that during the processes involved in the performance of the pupil's practical work, he should cultivate and develop in him the new and reliable sensory appreciation upon which a satisfactory standard of co-ordination depends.

To this end the mode of procedure is as follows: the teacher, having made his diagnosis of the cause or causes of the imperfections or defects which the pupil has developed in the incorrect use of himself, uses expert manipulation to give to the pupil the new sensory experiences required for the satisfactory use of the mechanisms concerned, the while giving him the correct guiding orders or directions which are the counterpart of the new sensory experiences which he is endeavouring to develop by means of his manipulation.

This procedure constitutes the *means whereby* the teacher makes it possible for the pupil to *prevent* (inhibition) the misdirected activities which are causing his psycho-physical imperfections. In this work the inhibitory process must take first place, and remain the primary factor in each and every new experience which is to be gained and become established during the cultivation and development of reliable sensory appreciation upon which a satisfactory standard of co-ordination depends.

With this aim in view, that is, the prevention of misdirected activities, the teacher from the outset carefully explains to the pupil that his part in this scheme is very different from that which is usually assigned to pupils under other teaching methods. He tells the pupil that, on receiving the directions or guiding orders, he must not attempt to carry them out; that, on the contrary, *he must inhibit the desire to do so in the case of each and every order which is given to him.* He must instead project the guiding orders as given to him whilst his teacher at the same time, by means of manipulation, will make the required readjustments and bring about the necessary co-ordinations, in this way performing for the pupils the particular movement or movements required, and giving him the new reliable sensory appreciation and the very best opportunity possible to connect the different guiding orders before attempting to put them into practice. This linking-up of the guiding orders or directions is all-important, for it is the counterpart of that linking-up of the parts of the organism which constitutes what we call co-ordination. The aim of re-education on a general basis is to bring about at all times and for all purposes, not a series of correct positions or postures, but *a co-ordinated use of the mechanisms in general.*

The second point to be noted in connexion with the technique we are advocating is that the directions or guiding orders given to the pupil are based in every case on the principle of ceasing to work in blind pursuit of an "end," and of attending instead to the *means whereby* this "end" can be attained. We have already considered this principle in its general application, but I am anxious to lay stress upon it again at this point, because it is of the utmost importance that the pupil should both accept this principle and apply it to his work in the sphere of re-education, for by no other method can he get the better of his old subconscious habits, and build up consciously the new and improved condition which he is anxious to bring about.

If we consider for a moment, we shall see the reason for this. For if the pupil thinks of a certain "end" as desirable and starts to pursue it directly, he will certainly take the course of action in regard to it that he has been accustomed to take in like conditions. In other words, he will follow his habitual procedure in regard to it, and should that procedure happen to be a bad one for the purpose (and the fact that he needs re-education proves this to be the case), he only strengthens the incorrect experiences in connexion with it by using this procedure again. If, on the other hand, the pupil *stops himself* from going to work in his usual way (inhibition), and proceeds to replace his old subconscious means by the new conscious means which his teacher has given him, and which he has therefore every reason to believe will bring about the desired result, he will have taken the first and most important step towards the breaking-down of a habit, and towards that constructive, conscious and reasoning control which tends towards a mastery of the situation.[1]

It is therefore impressed on the pupil from the beginning that, as the essential preliminary to any successful work on his part, *he*

---

[1] This applies equally to the breaking of habit in every sphere of activity.

*must refuse to work directly for his "end" and keep his attention entirely on the "means whereby" this end can be secured.*

In this way all responsibility for the final result is taken off the pupil. He has no "end" to work for, and therefore nothing to get right. All that is asked of him is, when he receives a guiding order, to *listen and wait;* to wait, because only by waiting can he be certain of preventing himself from relapsing into his old subconscious habits, and to listen, so that he learns to remember gradually and connect up the guiding orders which are the counterpart of the *means whereby* the teacher is employing to bring about the desired "end." In other words, he is asked to adopt consciously a principle of prevention as the basis of his practical work, and in every other way to leave the teacher a free hand.

## Chapter Three

# OUR MISTAKEN IDEAS
## ABOUT OURSELVES

Perhaps the most striking and at the same time the most pathetic instance of human delusion is to be found in the human creature's attitude towards his own psycho-physical defects, disadvantages, peculiarities, etc., on one hand, and towards his merits, advantages and natural gifts on the other. "To thine own self be true," is an inspiring incentive when the human creature's co-ordinated psycho-physical development has reached a point where that self cannot be duped by its sensations.

In connexion with unreliable sensory appreciation and with perverted ideas or conceptions of what is "right" or "wrong," where the human creature's uses of his own mechanisms are concerned, the following is a most significant illustration.

A little girl who had been unable to walk properly for some years was brought to the writer for a diagnosis of the defects in the use of the psycho-physical mechanisms which were responsible for her more or less crippled state. When this had been done, a request was made that a demonstration should be given to those present of the manipulative side of the work (the child, of course, to be the subject to be manipulated), so that certain readjustments and co-ordinations might be temporarily secured, thus shewing, in keeping with the diagnosis, the possibilities of re-education on a general basis in a case of this kind. The demonstration was successful from this point of view. For the time being the child's body was comparatively straightened out, that is, without the extreme twists and distortions that had been so noticeable when she came into the room. When this was done, the little girl looked across at her mother and said to her in an indescribable tone, "Oh! Mummie, he's pulled me *out of shape.*"

Here, indeed, is food for reflection for all who are concerned in any attempt to eradicate psycho-physical defects! In accordance with this poor little child's judgment, her crookedness was straightness, her sensory appreciation of her "out-of-shape" condition was

17

that it was "in shape." Imagine, then, what would be the result of her trying to get anything "right" by doing something herself, as she had always tried and had always been urged to try to do, whilst practising remedial exercises according to the directions and under the guidance of a teacher. Small wonder that all attempts to teach her had resulted in failure!

Consideration of the foregoing cannot but lead us to a full realization of what would have been the psycho-physical condition of such a child when she reached adolescence, if the orthodox methods of teaching in all spheres had been employed to help her. The child's remark is proof positive that, where her defects were concerned, her ideas and conceptions were dominated by her sensory appreciation, and that this sensory appreciation was not only unreliable but actually delusive. Her experiences in connexion with the functioning of her organism were consequently incorrect and harmful experiences, and as her judgment in these spheres was the result of these experiences, little wonder that her judgment of what was right and what wrong in her case was not only practically worthless, but constituted a positive danger to her future development. Unless in such cases a child is re-educated and co-ordinated on a basis of conscious control, it cannot acquire a new and reliable sensory appreciation, and, lacking this, it will grow up employing guiding sensations which are delusive and which tend to become more and more so with the advance of time. Incorrect experiences and bad judgment will be associated with this delusive guidance.

The first step then is to convince the pupil that his present misdirected activities are the result of incorrect conception and of imperfect sensory appreciation (feeling).

Now, in this regard, I would at once warn those who are inexperienced in this matter that the pupil, as a rule, will not be convinced on this point by discussion and argument alone. A pupil will, indeed, often assure his teacher that he sees the argument, and from his standpoint this statement may be true. But, in my experience, there is only one way by which a teacher can really convince a pupil that his sense of feeling is misleading him when he starts to carry out a movement, and that is *by demonstration upon the pupil's own organism.* A mirror should be used so that the pupil, as far as possible, can have ocular demonstration as well.

The next point of importance to be impressed upon the pupil is the necessity for listening carefully to the teacher's words, and for being quite clear as to the meaning that these words are intended to convey *before he attempts to act upon them.* This may seem a truism, but, as a matter of fact, it is at this point that we come up against a rock on which even a highly experienced teacher may make shipwreck. For, in every case, the pupil's conception of what his teacher is trying to convey to him by words *will be in accordance with his (the pupil's) psycho-physical make-up.*[1]

If, for instance, the pupil has fixed ideas in some particular direction, these fixed ideas must inevitably limit his capacity for "listening carefully" (a capacity which we are apt to take so much for granted), that is, for receiving the new ideas *as the teacher is trying to convey them to him.* In this connexion, therefore, a teacher in dealing with the shortcomings of a particular case must give due consideration to the pupil's fixed conceptions, otherwise these will greatly complicate the problem for both teacher and pupil. Certain of these fixed ideas are encountered in the case of almost every pupil; fixed ideas, for example, as to what constitutes the right and what the wrong method of going to work as a pupil; fixed ideas in regard to the necessity for concentration, if success is to attend the efforts of pupil and teacher; also a fixed belief (based on subconscious guidance) that, if a pupil is corrected for a defect, he should be taught *to do something* in order to correct it, instead of being taught, as a first principle, *how to prevent (inhibition) the wrong thing from being done.*

The teacher experienced in the work of re-education can diagnose at once, by the expression and use of the pupil's eyes, the degree of influence upon him of such conceptions, and at each step in the training he should take preventive measures to counteract this influence. It is absurd to try to teach a person who is in a more or less agitated or even anxious condition. We must have that calm condition which is characteristic of a person whose reasoning processes are operative.

The list of fixed conceptions given above might be increased a hundredfold. The peculiarities of fixed conceptions, like peculiari-

---

[1] In this sense it can be truly said that a pupil hears only what he wants to hear, because what he wants is decided by the standards fixed by his present habits.

ties of handwriting, differ greatly in different people, and the form they take depends, as in the case of handwriting again, upon the individual psycho-physical makeup.[1]

A teaching experience of over twenty-five years in a psycho-physical sphere has given me a very real knowledge of the psycho-physical difficulties which stand in the way of many adults who need re-education and co-ordination, and, as the result of this experience, I have no hesitation in stating that the pupil's fixed ideas and conceptions are the cause of the major part of his difficulties.

I will now take one of these fixed conceptions from my teaching experience, because it is so wide-spread and has such far-reaching and harmful effects upon life in general. I will talk about the habit which has become established in most pupils trained on a subconscious basis, and to which we have already referred, viz., *that of trying to correct one defect by doing something else, by "doing it right."*

Let us suppose that a person decides that he will take lessons in re-education from a certain teacher and comes for the first lesson. The teacher proceeds to indicate to the pupil, firstly, the results of his diagnosis of the pupil's psycho-physical peculiarities, delusions and defects which he proposes to attempt to eradicate; and, secondly, the *means whereby* the eradication is to be effected.

It invariably follows that by the time the teacher has concluded his statement, the pupil will have formed his own conception (often diametrically the reverse of his teacher's) of the facts disclosed, and unless he is a very unusual person, he will already have come to a decision in accordance with his preconceived ideas,

(1)  as to the cause or causes underlying the facts disclosed;
(2)  as to the ends that will be gained by the removal of these causes; and, most important of all,
(3)  as to the means he will adopt in order to gain these ends.

The present faulty subconscious use of the psycho-physical mechanism, in our educational and other spheres, makes for the

[1] All that is written here about fixed conceptions applies equally to the teacher as to the pupil.

gradual increase of defective equilibrium. It would seem that this fact is generally taken for granted, seeing that we expect defective equilibrium at a certain age, just as we expect the development of a flabby and protruding abdomen. This is surely the end of our contention that practice makes perfect; it also seems evident from this that there must be something wrong with the practice in the act of walking.

The fact is that people walk without any clear understanding of the guiding and controlling orders which command the satisfactory co-ordination and adjustment of the psycho-physical mechanism in the act of walking. Hence when one or more defects become present in the functioning of these mechanisms, even though the persons concerned may be aware of their cause or causes, they are incapable of establishing once more that standard of reliable sensory appreciation which would enable them to eradicate these defects. This needs a process of re-education on a general basis, which will restore satisfactory functioning throughout the organism, and so ensure a continued raising of the standard of psycho-physical equilibrium right on through life.

With almost every attempt to correct some supposed or real psycho-physical imperfection, new defects are developed which tend to lower the standard of psycho-physical equilibrium. In this connexion, it is an interesting but very unfortunate fact that this unsatisfactory condition develops in the subject hand in hand with the desire to hurry unduly, this being a subconscious endeavour to compensate for the growing lack of equilibrium and lack of control. In extreme cases of lack of equilibrium this manifestation is most pronounced. The subject becomes conscious, first, of a weakness or difficulty which affects his general equilibrium in walking, and, without making any attempt to discover the cause or causes of this newly recognized weakness or difficulty, proceeds, as he would put it, to try to "walk properly," *i.e.,* to walk without the slight unsteadiness of which he is conscious. But the fact that this weakness or difficulty has developed is proof that the subject's guiding sensations and general psycho-physical co-ordinations of the organism are defective. It is therefore obvious that any subconsciously directed efforts on his part to "walk properly," *i.e.,* more steadily, will be carried out according to these same defective guiding sensations and imperfectly co-ordinated mechanisms, and cannot therefore succeed.

It must be remembered that during all these "trial-and-error" experiences the fear reflexes are being unduly excited by the fear of falling, and by the general unreliability and uncertainty of the psycho-physical processes which are employed during such subconsciously directed efforts. Taking this process as a whole, we shall find that most harmful psycho-physical conditions will be developed, which soon manifest themselves in other spheres of psychophysical functioning, and very often culminate at last in some serious crisis.

It is easy to trace the development of this lack of equilibrium in what is usually considered the "purely physical" sphere. Let us take by way of illustration the case of a boy who, in the ordinary way, would be classed as a good walker. We will assume that he has been injured at the age of, say, thirteen by being thrown from a horse or by a fall downstairs, or has met with some other accident which has necessitated his being treated by a doctor and being confined to his bed for some time. It is obvious that his injury and the cessation of his ordinary activities will produce in the patient a more or less weakened condition generally, and also definite specific difficulties in connexion with the injured parts of the organism. The result is that at the psychological moment when the patient makes the first attempt to resume walking, certain impeding factors will manifest themselves which he will immediately proceed to overcome by "trying to walk properly" as he understands it. His attempt to walk "properly" must necessarily be on the subconscious plan of "trial-and-error," for it is almost certain that he has never known HOW he walked, never had the least idea of the guiding orders concerned with the co-ordinations essential to the act of walking and to the development of satisfactory equilibrium.[1]

---

[1] My reader will probably think of the case of some friend who has made an attempt to "walk properly" after an injury, and who is now walking about to HIS OWN satisfaction. My point is, that the subject is not capable of judging whether his use of his psycho-physical mechanisms in walking is satisfactory or not. It is quite certain that anyone with an expert knowledge in this connexion could point to certain harmful defects in the subject's use of himself which are the combined result of the injury, the varied experiences in treatment and recovery, and the attempts "to walk," all of which are indicative of comparative weakness, a sense of interference with equilibrium and a general loss of control.

It will be necessary here to analyse the psycho-physical processes involved in his effort, for success in such efforts demands a high standard of co-ordinated functioning of the organism. Experience has proved to us that this standard of functioning is not at the command of a person who has been through the experiences connected with such an injury, and with the subsequent treatment and gradual recovery to the point when what we call the convalescent stage has been reached. Real success is practically impossible and for the reasons which follow.

These attempts to walk would be made at a time when the subject was conscious of a weakness throughout the whole organism, of a comparative loss of control, of an interference with the psycho-physical equilibrium, of a lack of confidence, together with a whole series of hopes and fears in regard to what he will or will not be able to do, associated, again, with fears which have their origin in the pain which results from his incorrect subconscious attempts to use parts that have been injured. This whole combination of psycho-physical conditions constitutes a set of experiences which are new as compared with those present at the time of the accident. Each subconscious attempt to walk awakens consciousness of shortcomings, of strange and often alarming sensations, and tends to increase the real difficulties, viz., those concerned with that correct use of the psycho-physical organism in general upon which "walking properly" depends.

It will thus be clear that the attempt to walk properly by subconscious guidance would merely be an attempt to revert to the habit or habits established in the act of walking before the accident. This way of walking was instinctive, and a particular instinctive process is the result of certain psycho-physical conditions operating, as we say, by instinct. Change those conditions quickly and you interfere with the reliability of the working of the particular instinct.

This illustration furnishes us with a splendid practical instance of a definite need calling for new experiences in psycho-physical use. The boy wishes to walk. The stimulus to do so produces an immediate response involving the processes concerned with subconscious guidance and control which are habitual, but which depend for efficiency upon a given standard of co-ordinated functioning of the organism. Unfortunately, this standard has been lowered by his experiences associated with the accident, and the psycho-physical machinery does not work as satisfactorily as before; in fact, in the majority of such cases, it works very unsatisfactorily. The subject is able to compare the result of his present efforts with those he made before his injury. They compare very badly, and he is conscious of the fact. This merely causes him to "try harder," as he would put it, "to walk properly," and, on a subconscious basis, he has no alternative but to continue the unintelligent method of "trial-and-error."

We will now outline the experiences which the procedure based on the principles of re-education on a conscious general basis would have ensured in the foregoing case. In the first place, we should not allow the subject to try to "walk properly" until he had been given, by expert manipulation, correct experiences in the general use of the psycho-physical mechanisms, and had become well acquainted with the correct guiding and controlling orders which would assist in the securing of the *means whereby* he should use the mechanisms in any attempt to walk properly.

The recognition of weakness or difficulty would be the signal for an examination of the psycho-physical mechanisms involved in the use of the organism as a whole, which in turn would enable us to note the defects and peculiarities in the use of these mechanisms in the specific act of walking. The technique we advocate would demand in practice that the subject should cease to try to improve his walking. We would therefore endeavour to convince him by demonstration that his efforts to improve his walking by "muddling through by instinct" are not only futile but quite absurd. By the same process (demonstration) he would be shewn that as soon as he receives the stimulus to walk, he must begin his remedial work by employing his inhibitory powers to prevent the use of the wrong subconscious guidance and direction associated with his conception of "walking." In this connexion it is explained to him that it is the use of the incorrect, subconscious guiding orders to the mechanisms concerned with the act of walking, associated with unreliable sensory appreciation, which has caused the mechanisms to be used imperfectly, resulting in the weakness and difficulties with which we are contending.

When the subject is more or less familiar with these inhibitory experiences, we go on to give him a knowledge of the new and correct directive and guiding orders which, with the aid of manipulation, are to bring about the satisfactory use of the mechanisms in a sitting, prone, or other position. These experiences must be repeated until the new and reliable sensory appreciation becomes established, by which time there will have taken place an actual change in the use of the psycho-physical mechanisms of the organism in general, making for a satisfactory condition of co-ordination and adjustment. When the required improvement in the general co-ordinations and adjustments has been secured, the processes we have outlined will be more or less in conscious operation, and a corresponding improvement in equilibrium in walking will be the result.

The reader must understand that the details involved in such processes (differing as these do in each case) cannot be set forth here, and that, moreover, from the very first lessons the teacher's aim would be to cause the pupil to be conscious of what he should or should NOT do, and to give such help to the pupil as would enable him to begin at once to apply the principles involved, not only to his attempts at walking, but more or less to all the acts of his daily life. In other words, the pupil is not taught to perform certain new exercises or to assume new postures for a given time each day, whilst continuing to use his faulty mechanisms and unreliable guiding sensations in his old way during his other activities, but he is shewn HOW he may at once check, more or less, the faulty use of these mechanisms in the general activities of his daily life.

An increase in lack of equilibrium in what is called the "physical" sphere, will be found, in every case, to go hand in hand with a corresponding lack of equilibrium in so-called "mental" spheres. And in any consideration of "mental" and "physical" phenomena, it must be remembered that in our present stage of evolution on the subconscious plane, the response to any stimulus or stimuli is at least seventy-five per cent subconscious response (chiefly feeling) as against twenty-five per cent any other response, this estimate of the ratio of subconscious response being probably too low.

*Chapter Four*

# A CASE HISTORY: THE STUTTERER

I will now consider the case of a man with an impediment in his speech who was sent to me for advice and help. He told me that he had taken lessons from specialists who treated speech defects, and had done his best to carry out their instructions and to practise their exercises. He had always had special difficulty with sounds which called for the use of the tongue and lips, particularly with the consonants T and D, but although he had been more or less successful in doing the exercises themselves, his stutter was as bad as ever in ordinary conversation, especially when he was hurried or excited.

As is my custom with a new pupil, I noted specially the way he walked into my room and sat down in a chair, and it was obvious to me that his general use of himself was more than usually harmful. When he spoke, I also noticed a wrong use of his tongue and lips and certain defects in the use of his head and neck, involving undue depression of the larynx and undue tension of the face and neck muscles. I then pointed out to him that his stutter was not an isolated symptom of wrong use confined to the organs of speech, but that it was associated with other symptoms of wrong use and functioning in other parts of his organism.

As he doubted this, I went on to explain that I had been able to demonstrate to every stutterer who had come to me for help that he "stuttered" with many other different parts of his body besides his tongue and lips. "Usually," I said, "these other defects remain unobserved or ignored until they reach the point where the wrong functioning manifests itself in some form of so-called 'physical' or 'mental' disorder. In your case, your stutter interferes with your work and hinders intercourse with your fellows, and so you have not been able to ignore it, but this may well turn out to be a blessing in disguise if it is the means of making you aware, before too late, of the other more serious defects which I have pointed out to you, and which will tend, as time goes on, to become more and more exaggerated." I assured him that my long years of practical experience in dealing with the difficulties and idiosyncrasies of people who stutter had convinced me that stuttering was one of the most interesting specific symptoms of a general cause, namely, misdirection of the use of the psycho-physical mechanisms, and I did not wish to take him as a pupil, unless he was prepared to work with me on the basis of correcting this misdirection of use generally, as the primary step in remedying his defects in speech. I could promise him, however, that if he decided to come to me and I was successful in making certain changes for the better in his manner of using his mechanisms, a change for the better would also come about in the functioning of his organism, and his stuttering would tend to disappear in the process. He saw the point and decided to take lessons.

I began by pointing out to him various outstanding symptoms of his wrong habitual use, one of the most marked of these being the undue amount of muscle tension that he was in the habit of employing throughout his organism whenever he tried to speak. This extreme muscle tension was an impeding factor in the functioning of his mechanisms generally, and rendered impossible a satisfactory use of his tongue and lips, and the more he tried by any special effort of "will" to speak without stuttering, the more certain he was to increase the already undue muscle tension and so to defeat his own end.

The reason for this, I explained to him, was that he did not start to speak until he had brought about the amount of tension which was associated with his habitual use and which caused him to *feel that he could speak;* i.e., he would decide that the moment had come for him to speak only when his *feeling* told him that he was using his mechanisms to the best advantage, and this moment, in the last analysis, was when his sensory appreciation (the only guide he had as to the amount of muscle tension necessary) registered to him as "right" the amount of tension which he habitually employed in speaking and which was therefore familiar to him.

Unfortunately, the familiar amount of tension that "felt right" to him was the unnecessary amount associated with the wrong habitual use of his mechanisms of which his stuttering was a symptom, and I therefore urged him to recognize from the begin-

ning that the "feeling," upon which he was relying to tell him
when his use was right for speaking, was untrustworthy as a register of muscle tension, and that he must not depend upon it for
guidance in his attempts to speak. How, I asked him, could he expect to judge by his feeling the amount of tension he should employ
in speaking, when he was unfamiliar with the sensory experience
of speaking with the due amount? Obviously, he could not "know"
a sensation he had never experienced, and as sensory experience
cannot be conveyed by the spoken word, no amount of telling on
my part could convey to him the unfamiliar sensory experience of
speaking with less tension and without stuttering. The only way to
convince him that he could speak with a less amount of muscle
tension would be to give him this unfamiliar experience.

(1)  the directions for the inhibition of the wrong habitual use
     of his mechanisms associated with the excessive muscle
     tension;
(2)  the directions for the employment of the primary control
     leading to a new and improved use which would be asso-
     ciated with a due amount of muscle tension.

I then asked him to project these directions whilst I with my
hands gave him the new sensory experiences of use corresponding
to these directions, in order that the trustworthiness of his sensory
appreciation in relation to the use of his mechanisms might be
gradually restored, and that by this means he might in time acquire
a register of the due amount of tension required for speaking, as
distinct from the undue amount of tension associated with his
stuttering.

I continued this procedure, until I had repeated for him the new
sensory experiences of use often enough to justify me in allowing
him to attempt to employ his new "means-whereby" for speaking
and for saying the words and consonants that caused him special
difficulty.

It is impossible in the space at my command to put down all
the details of the variations of the teacher's art that were employed
to bring my pupil to this point, for a teacher's technique naturally
varies in detail according to the particular needs and difficulties

of each pupil. Those of my readers, however, who have followed the account of the difficulties I encountered when I first attempted to employ the new "means-whereby" in my reciting, will be able to realize the kind of difficulty we were faced with all along, when I say that my pupil was a confirmed "end-gainer."

At the beginning of this new stage in our work together I reminded him how his progress up to this point had been hampered by his habit of end-gaining and of "trying to be right," and I warned him that unless he succeeded in side-stepping it, he would have little chance of applying his new "means-whereby" to his difficulties in speaking, for if, at the critical moment of starting to say a difficult word, he still went directly for his end and tried to say the word in the way that "felt right" to him, he would be bound to revert to his old habitual use in speaking and so stutter.

Events proved how difficult it was for my pupil to take practical heed of this warning. I would repeatedly urge him, whenever I gave him a sound or word to pronounce, always to inhibit his old habitual response to my request by refusing to attempt to pronounce the sound or word until he had taken time to think out and employ the new directions for the use which he had decided upon as best for his purpose. He would agree to do this, but as soon as I asked him to pronounce some sound or word, he would fail to inhibit his response to the stimulus of my voice, and forgetting all about the new directions he had been asked to employ, he would immediately try to repeat the sound, with the result that he was at once dominated by his old habits of use associated with the extreme muscle tension that *felt right* to him, and so stuttered as badly as ever.[1] In short, his very desire to "be right in gaining his end" defeated the end.

In every stutterer of whom I have had experience this habit of reacting too quickly to stimuli is always associated with sensory untrustworthiness, undue muscle tension and misdirection of energy, but in this pupil's case the habit of going directly for his end, and of trying to "feel right" in doing it, had been positively cultivated in him by the methods employed by his previous teachers in trying to "cure" his stutter.

---

[1] In order that the reader should not think this difficulty was peculiar to this pupil, I wish to state that I have had similar experiences with all my pupils. How could it be otherwise when "end-gaining" is a universal habit?

It would appear that the "end-gaining" principle underlies every one of the exercises given by teachers who, whether by orthodox or unorthodox methods, deal with stuttering as a specific defect, and I will take as an example the exercises that had been given to my pupil to meet his special difficulty in pronouncing words beginning with T or D.

His former teachers had recognized that the use of his tongue and lips was unsatisfactory for the purpose of pronouncing these consonants, and in order to overcome the difficulty had instructed him to practice certain exercises involving the use of these specific parts in saying T or D.

Now this procedure could only aggravate the difficulty, for the idea of trying to say T or D acted as an incentive to the pupil to employ the habitual use of himself associated with the wrong use of his tongue and lips. As long as this wrong habitual use remained unchanged, this association persisted and he had little chance of getting rid of this incentive, so that to ask him under these conditions to practice saying T and D as a remedy for his stuttering was tantamount to giving him an added incentive to stutter.

This was borne out by what I observed when he shewed me how he had been practicing these exercises. I watched him closely and saw that as soon as he started to do them, he at once made an undue amount of tension generally, continued to increase the tension of the muscles of the lips, cheeks and tongue, and tried to say T and D before his tongue had taken up the best position for the purpose. This attempt was as bound to result in failure as would be the attempt of a motorist to change gears before the clutch has done its work in getting the cogs into the position in which they will mesh. It was evident that he had been trying in all his practice in the past to gain his end without being in command of the means whereby this end could be successfully gained, and the fact that the majority of these attempts had been unsuccessful had brought him to a state of lack of confidence in himself, which added considerably to the difficulty of breaking his "end-gaining" habit.

As far as I am aware, all methods of "curing" stuttering, however they may differ in detail, are all based on the same "end-gaining" principle. The adviser will select some symptom or symptoms as the cause of his pupil's stuttering and will give him specific instructions or exercises to help him.

I am well aware that it has proved possible by such methods to stop people from stuttering, but I would question the common assumption that because this is so, a genuine "cure" has been effected. For in cases where it is claimed that a stutter has been "cured," there is usually something peculiar or hesitating about the manner of speaking, and those concerned do not seem in the least perturbed that the harmful conditions of undue muscle tension, misdirection of energy and untrustworthiness of sensory appreciation, present in the case when the "cure" was begun, are still in evidence now that what is considered a successful "cure" has been brought about.

No method of "cure" can be accepted as effective or scientific, if, in the process of removing certain selected symptoms, other symptoms have been left untouched and if new, unwished-for symptoms have appeared. If this test is applied to a stutterer after he has been "cured" by such methods, it will be found too often that the original defects of undue muscular tension, misdirection of energy and untrustworthiness of sensory appreciation have been increased in the process of the "cure."

I admit that these defects may not bring about a recurrence of the stutter, but even so, they are almost certain to lead to the further development of other undesirable symptoms which constantly remain unrecognized. This invariably happens when defects and diseases are "cured" by specific methods, and explains why, in spite of the immense number of "cures" recorded, the troubles in the human organism would seem to be increasing and calling for more and more "cures."

It is important to remember that there is a working balance in the use of all the parts of the organism, and that for this reason the use of the specific part (or parts) in any activity can influence the use of the other parts, and vice versa. Under instinctive direction this working balance becomes habitual and "feels right," and the point at which the influence of the use of any part will make itself felt will vary and the influence of the particular use be strong or weak according to the nature of the stimulus of the end activity desired. If a defect is recognized in the use of a part, and an attempt is made to correct this defect by changing the use of the part without bringing about at the same time a corresponding change in the use of the other parts, the habitual working balance in the use of the whole will be disturbed. Unless, therefore, the person attempting to make a change in the use of a specific part has an understanding of what is required to bring about at the same time a corresponding change in the use of the other parts which will make for a satisfactory working balance and therefore be complementary to the new use that he is trying to bring about at one point, one of two things is bound to happen:

either,

(1)   the stimulus of the desire to gain his end, by means of the old use associated with the habitual working balance which "feels right," will be so strong that it will dominate the stimulus to cultivate a new and improved use of a certain part associated with an unfamiliar working balance which "feels wrong";

or,

(2)   if the change in the use of a part is made in the face of impeding factors in the use of the other parts (as happens in any specific method of treatment employed to correct a defect in a part), the working balance between the use of that part and the use of all the other parts will be so thrown out of gear that the use of the other parts will be adversely affected in their turn, and new defects in the use of these parts developed.

After my pupil had shewn me the exercises he had been told to do, I explained to him that in practicing them he had been indulging in his old wrong habits of general use of himself, and thereby actually *cultivating* the wrong habits of use of his tongue and lips which had made him stutter. I impressed upon him once more that if he wished ever to be confident of saying T and D and words in which these consonants occur without stuttering, *he must refuse to respond to any stimulus either from within or without to say T or D;* in other words, whenever the idea of saying T or D came to him, he must inhibit his desire to try and say it correctly, until he had learned what use of his tongue and lips was required in his case for saying T or D without stuttering, and until he could put into practice the necessary directions for this new use of his tongue and lips *whilst continuing to give the directions for the primary control of the new and improved use of himself generally.*

He understood the reason for this, but his attempts at coöperating with me proved more or less unsuccessful for some time. Over and over again I got him to the point where the use of his tongue and lips in association with his general use was such that I knew he could pronounce T and D without the undue muscle tension that made him stutter, but when at this point I asked him to repeat one of the sounds, he would either

(1)  forget to inhibit his old response, change back to his old conditions of use and increase the tension to the point when he *felt* that he could say T or D, try to say it in this way and stutter, or

(2)  on the occasions when he remembered to inhibit his old response and to employ the new "means-whereby" for saying T and D without stuttering, he would make no attempt to repeat the sound.

In both these cases he was actuated by the same motive. He associated the act of speaking, especially the pronunciation of consonants that were difficult for him, with a given amount of muscle tension, and as I have already shewn, he had come to believe that it was impossible for him to speak until he *felt* this undue amount of tension. This explains why he made no attempt to speak until he had deliberately brought about the familiar but excessive tension which caused him to stutter. In this way he simply reinforced the old sensory experiences of undue muscle tension already associated with his habitual use, and with his habit of trying to *feel right* in gaining his end.

To deal with this difficulty I made a point of giving my pupil day after day the experience of receiving a stimulus to gain a certain end and of remembering to refuse to gain that end, since this refusal meant that at one fell swoop he inhibited all the wrong habits of use associated with his habitual way of gaining that end. In proportion as he was successful in inhibiting his immediate response to any stimulus, he became able to defeat his desire to gain his ends in the way that felt right to him, and *as long as he continued this inhibition,* I on my side was able to repeat for him, until they became familiar, the new sensory experiences associated with an improved general use of his mechanisms, including the right use of his tongue and lips. By continuing to cooperate with me on these lines, he gradually acquired sufficient experience in the direction of this new use to be able to employ it successfully as the "means-whereby" of pronouncing the consonants which had caused him special difficulty.

But, more important than this, my pupil in the course of this procedure had learned that if he inhibited his immediate instinctive reaction to any stimulus to "do," he could prevent the misdirection of his use and the associated undue muscle tension which had been the marked feature of all his reactions to stimuli, and which had hampered him not only in his speaking but in all his activities, both "physical" and "mental," and if he chose to apply this principle to his activities in other spheres, he would have at his command a means of controlling the nature of his reaction to stimuli, that is, of acquiring a control of what is called "conscious behavior."[1]

Certain features of this pupil's case occur with practically every pupil.

[1] The following is of interest in this connexion. One of my pupils has just told me that before he came to me for lessons he used to have uncontrollable fits of temper, but that since having the work he has no trouble in that way, and that all his family notice the change. He asked me to explain how it was that what he looked upon as a "nervous" or "mental" symptom could be affected by the kind of work I was doing with him. In reply I asked him how other people knew when he had lost his temper, and he answered that they would know by the tone of his voice, the expression of his face, the look in his eyes, or by his gestures and excited manner generally. I then asked him how these reactions could be possible except through the use of what he thought of as his "physical" self. For instance, the voice must be used if we are to judge its tone, there must be use of the eyes if they are to flash, of the muscles of the face for change of expression, and, for excitability to be manifested the whole of the mechanisms of use must be stimulated into undue activity and muscle tension.

Change the manner of use and you change the conditions throughout the organism; the old reaction associated with the old manner of use and the old conditions cannot therefore take place, for the means are no longer there. In other words, the old habitual reflex activity has been changed and will not recur. If loss of control can be manifested only by means of the use of ourselves, it follows that a conscious direction of an improving use will bring us for the first time within striking distance of a conscious control of human reaction or behaviour.

During the earlier stages of a pupil's lessons when the use of his mechanisms is still unsatisfactory, I have constantly found that he fails to inhibit the old instinctive direction of his use, with the result that his directions for the new use do not become operative. Before I can get a chance to help him, he proceeds to gain his end in accordance with his habitual wrong use, and it is practically impossible under these circumstances to stop him from gaining his end in this way.

On the other hand, when he has learned at a later stage in his lessons to inhibit the instinctive direction of his use and the directions for the new use have become operative, so that I am enabled to give him the corresponding sensory experiences, I have found that although he now has at his command the best conditions possible for gaining his end, he will not make any attempt to gain it. He cannot believe that the end can be gained with these improved conditions present; they "feel so wrong," as he puts it, that he instinctively refuses to employ them.

When this difficulty arises, it is necessary for me to give him the actual experience of gaining his end by what he feels is a wrong use of his mechanisms, and when I have succeeded in doing this, he invariably remarks how much easier the new way is than the old way, and how much less effort it requires. Yet in spite of this admission, the actual experience of gaining his end in this new way has to be repeated for him again and again before the improved use "feels right" to him, and before he gains the necessary confidence in employing it.

The lesson to be learned from all this is that since our particular way of reacting to stimuli is in accordance with our familiar habits of use, the incentive to try to gain any given end is inextricably bound up with this familiar use. This explains why, if a pupil's familiar use is changed to one that is unfamiliar and therefore unassociated with his habitual way of reacting to stimuli, he has little or no incentive to gain that given end. As long as the conditions of use and the associated feeling are wrong in a person, the incentive to gain a given end by the familiar wrong use appears to be almost irresistible, but when these conditions have been changed to conditions which are best for the purpose of gaining the end, there seems to be practically no incentive to gain it.

This is not surprising, for when a person's sensory appreciation of his use is wrong and his belief as to what he can or cannot do is based on what he feels, gaining an end by a use that is unfamiliar means for him taking a plunge in the dark. Even when I have explained to a pupil why this difficulty has arisen in his case, and he understands the reason for it "intellectually," he will need, more often than not, considerable encouragement and practical assistance in order to be enabled to make the experience of gaining a given end by means of a use that is new and unfamiliar to him. Once this has been done for him, however, he becomes conscious of a new experience that he is desirous to repeat, and repetition of this experience in time convinces him that his previous beliefs and judgments in this connexion were wrong. As a result there gradually develops in him an incentive to employ the new use, and this becomes at last far stronger than the incentive to employ the old use, for its development is the outcome of a reasoned procedure which he finds he can consciously direct and control with a confidence he has never before experienced.

One of the most remarkable of man's characteristics is his capacity for becoming used to conditions of almost any kind, whether good or bad, both in the self and in the environment, and once he has become used to such conditions they seem to him both right and natural. This capacity is a boon when it enables him to adapt himself to conditions which are desirable, but it may prove a great danger when the conditions are undesirable. When his sensory appreciation is untrustworthy, it is possible for him to become so familiar with seriously harmful conditions of misuse of himself that these malconditions will feel right and comfortable.

My teaching experience has shewn me that the worse these conditions are in a pupil and the longer they have been in existence, the more familiar and right they feel to him and the harder it is to teach him how to overcome them, no matter how much he may wish to do so. In other words, his ability to learn a new and more satisfactory use of himself is, as a rule, in inverse ratio to the degree of misuse present in his organism and the duration of these harmful conditions.

This point must be understood and taken into practical consideration by anyone forming a plan of procedure for improving the use and functioning of the mechanisms throughout the organism as a means of eradicating defects, peculiarities and bad habits.

Towards the end of his lessons my pupil asked me why it should be so much more difficult to overcome the habit of stuttering than the habit of over-smoking. He then went on to tell me that at one time he had been an inveterate smoker, but realizing that the habit was getting too much of a hold on him, he had decided he must give it up. He had first tried the plan of reducing the number of cigarettes he smoked per day, but as he found that he could not keep within the prescribed limit, he had decided that the only way for him to succeed in breaking his habit was to give up smoking altogether. He put this decision into practice and had become a non-smoker. He now wanted to know why his efforts to overcome his stuttering had not been equally successful.

I pointed out to him that the two habits presented very different problems.

The smoker can abstain from smoking without interrupting the necessary activities of his daily life, and as the temptation to smoke to excess results, as every chain-smoker knows, from the fact that each pipe, cigar or cigarette smoked acts as a stimulus to the smoking of another, every time he abstains from smoking he is breaking a link in the chain.

The stutterer, on the other hand, cannot abstain from speaking because his daily intercourse with his fellows depends on it. Every time he speaks, therefore, he is thrown into the way of temptation to indulge in his familiar wrong habits of use of his vocal organs, tongue and lips, and so to stutter. The stimulus to speak is one that he cannot evade in the way a smoker can evade the stimulus to smoke if he so wills it, so that the habit of stuttering calls for a much more fundamental form of control.

Satisfactory control of the act of speaking demands a satisfactory standard of the general use of the mechanisms, since the satisfactory use of the tongue and lips and the required standard of control of the respiratory and vocal organs depend upon this satisfactory general use. This being so, the unsatisfactory general use of the mechanisms which, as we have seen, is present in every stutterer, constitutes a formidable obstacle in the way of mastering his habit.

The situation is very different for the smoker, for the act of smoking does not demand any such high standard of use of the mechanisms, and although unsatisfactory conditions of use are frequently present in his case, the influence which they exercise in preventing him from overcoming his particular habit is small in comparison.

Still another element enters into the case. The habit which the smoker is trying to overcome is one which he has himself developed in the process of satisfying a desire. The stutterer, on the other hand, is dealing with a habit which has not been developed in the process of satisfying a desire, but which has gradually grown to become part of the use of the mechanisms which he habitually employs for all the activities of his daily life. This explains why the smoking habit is relatively superficial and in this degree easier to overcome, and why my pupil had been able *by himself* to solve the problem of his over-smoking, but had not been able to deal with his habit of stuttering without the help of a teacher who understood how to give him the means whereby he could *himself* command that satisfactory use of his mechanisms generally which includes the correct use of the tongue, lips and vocal organs for the act of speaking.

I would emphasize here that the process of eradicating any such defect as stuttering by these means makes the greatest demands on the time, patience and skill of both teacher and pupil, since, as we have seen, it calls for

(1) the inhibition of the instinctive direction of energy associated with familiar sensory experiences of wrong habitual use, and

(2) the building up in its place of a conscious direction of energy through the repetition of unfamiliar sensory experiences associated with new and satisfactory use.

This process of directing energy out of familiar into new and unfamiliar paths, as a means of changing the manner of reacting to stimuli, implies of necessity an ever-increasing ability on the part of both teacher and pupil to "pass from the known to the unknown." It is therefore a process which is true to the principle involved in all human growth and development.

## Chapter Five

# ABOUT BREATHING

We shall probably find the best practical illustration of the need for correct sensory experiences in guidance and control if we consider sensory appreciation in its connexion with the psycho-mechanics of respiration. It is universally admitted that there are harmful defects in the use of the respiratory mechanisms and a corresponding deterioration in the chest capacity and mobility of the great majority of people. The scientific medical man describes certain types of children as born with a "low respiratory need," and this really means that when the child is born, it is more or less imperfectly co-ordinated and its organism is functioning much nearer to its minimum than to its maximum capacity. This condition of inadequate vital functioning is present in the greater number of men, women, and children of today, and is one that is commonly associated with what we speak of as "bad breathing." For we say that a person is a "bad breather," or that he "breathes imperfectly." But we must remember that this so-called "bad breathing" is only a symptom and not a primary cause of his malcondition, for the standard of breathing depends upon the standard of general co-ordinated use of the psycho-physical mechanisms. What we ought to say, therefore, in such a case is not that a person "breathes badly," but that he is badly co-ordinated. The truth is that when we refer to this mal-co-ordinated condition as "bad breathing," we are mistaking a general malcondition for a specific defect, and the conception of the respiratory act which makes this error possible, and which affects even our way of expressing it, provides yet another instance of the dominance of our general attitude by the "end-gaining" principle.

This "end-gaining" principle is again dominant when it is decided that a person who is spoken of as a "bad breather" needs specific "breathing exercises" or "lessons in breathing." We shall see that in this, as in so many other spheres, a vicious circle is developed.

In the attempt to make this clear we must give consideration

41

to the fundamental principles upon which these breathing exercises (usually called "deep-breathing" exercises) or "lessons in breathing" are based. Take any book on breathing, whether written by a scientific author or by an expert in vocal or "physical culture," and read the written instructions in connexion with the exercises therein advocated. Take the opportunity also, when possible, to be present when the unfortunate children or adults in a gymnasium are being given a lesson in breathing or are performing their breathing exercises. You will then have proof that the whole of the processes concerned are directed towards specific and not general improvement, and though the people who are guilty of teaching "breathing exercises" may differ in detail of method, they all base their work alike on the same specific "end-gaining" principle. I shall now proceed to detail the processes involved.

The pupil is asked to take a deep breath. He may also be asked to perform some "physical" movement at the same time as he takes the deep breath, the idea behind this request being that the performance of the movement may help to increase the chest expansion. Yet it is a scientific fact that all "physical" tension tends to cause thoracic (chest) rigidity and breathlessness (lack of respiratory control), two conditions which should be avoided as far as possible by such pupils during their attempts to pass from conditions which are symptomatic of bad breathing to those which ensure satisfactory respiratory functioning.

It will be necessary for the layman to watch the pupil (or pupils) carefully during their attempts to carry out their written or spoken instructions in connexion with "deep breathing." Here we wish to refer only to the defective *general* use of the psycho-physical organism during these attempts. In order to make the point, we must refer to the fact that the pupil or the teacher, or both, must have recognized certain harmful manifestations which called for some remedial procedure on the lines of "deep-breathing," etc. Hence the decision to employ "deep-breathing" as a remedy. These harmful manifestations would be the result of certain incorrect psycho-physical uses of the organism. This would indicate that the sensory appreciation in the sphere of guidance and control of the psycho-physical mechanisms concerned must have become unreliable and defective, and in the present instance, so far as the observation of the teacher and pupil is concerned, certain defects must have been particularly noticeable in the use of the breathing mechanisms.

Here we have a clear case of certain established incorrect uses of the mechanisms, associated with a condition of unreliable sensory guidance and control, and any effort to remedy these incorrect uses by means of such processes as "deep-breathing" or "lessons in breathing" is merely an attempt to correct a *general* defective condition of psycho-mechanics by a *specific* remedial process. In other words, it is an attempt to correct the imperfect uses by the performance of exercises, the guidance and direction in such performance being associated with the same imperfect sensory appreciation which was already established when the lessons began. This means that with the continued practice of the exercises, the original defects in the general use of the mechanisms will become more and more pronounced and, what is more, increase in number.

It may be argued that, as the result of the lessons, the pupil's chest measurements are increased, that he "feels better," and so on. We are quite ready to admit that this may be so, but owing to the unreliability of his sensory appreciation, what he feels is as likely as not to be a delusion. Of what avail, therefore, is it for the pupil to "feel better," if he is still left with a defective sensory appreciation to guide him in all his activities during his waking moments as well as his sleeping hours? It is only a matter of time before the unfortunate pupil will be awakened from his dream by discovering that he has developed certain other serious conditions. I should like here to point out that these serious conditions must result, sooner or later, from the lack in such cases of a reliable guiding sensory appreciation, also from the lack of psycho-physical co-ordination which is associated therewith, and which continues to increase whilst these conditions are present. We have all known people who tell of the improvement in their chest measurement from the practice of exercises. The writer has examined many such in the course of thirty years' professional investigation. In the majority of these cases, the supposed increase in chest capacity has been chiefly due to muscular development on the outside of the bony chest, in other cases to some distortion or distortions cultivated during the process involved, rather than to that co-ordinated use of the psycho-physical system which is associated with a real increase in the intrathoracic (inner chest) capacity.[1] And it is the same in the case of those who tell you that they "feel better" as the result of these exercises, for to the expert observer it is obvious that the habit of "sniffing" (sucking in air), the contraction of the alae nasi, the depression of the larynx, and all the accompanying defective use of the organism associated with the practice of the exercises must, sooner or later, cause serious nose, ear, eye, and throat troubles. In other words, the exponents of these breathing exercises act in direct pursuance of their "end," remaining oblivious to the harmfulness of the *means whereby* they are attempting to bring this "end" about, and to the many wrong uses they are cultivating during the process.

This method of procedure, as we have seen, is the very opposite of that which underlies the process of re-education, readjustment and co-ordination on a conscious, general basis, and we will consider the application of this process to a satisfactory use of the psycho-physical mechanisms.

We will begin by a consideration of the fundamental psycho-physical principles underlying the act of breathing. In the course of this consideration it will be found that breathing is many times removed from the primary principle concerned, and that, therefore, it is incorrect and harmful to speak of "teaching a person to breathe," or of "giving lessons in breathing or deep-breathing." Such a stimulus to the subconsciously controlled person at once induces projections of all the established incorrect guiding orders associated with imperfect or inadequate breathing processes; in other words, this stimulus sets in motion all our bad habits in breathing.

Breathing is that psycho-physical act by means of which air is taken into and expelled from the lungs of the creature. The lungs are an extremely interesting part of our anatomy. They consist of two bags containing a net-work of cells capable of contraction and expansion, with air passages and blood vessels so associated and constituted that the oxygen contained in the air, when taken into

---

[1] An interesting delusion prevalent with teachers of breathing exercises is that of mistaking an increase in the muscle development on the outer walls of the chest for increase in intra-chest (thoracic) capacity.

the lungs, can be absorbed through the tissue of the blood vessels and cells and air passages, whilst carbonic acid gas (poison) passes through this tissue from the blood-vessels into the lung cells to be expelled from the lungs. The thorax (chest) has a bony structure, made up of the vertebrae of the spine, the different ribs and the sternum (breast-bone), those ribs which are attached to the sternum as well as to the spine being much less mobile than those which are not attached to the sternum, the most mobile being known as "floating ribs." The lungs are enclosed within the cavity of this bony thorax of which the diaphragm is the floor, and the only entrance to which is through the trachea (windpipe). From the very first breath there is a more or less constant air pressure (atmospheric pressure) within the lungs, but not any air pressure on the outside of the lungs. Air pressure is sufficient to overcome the elasticity of the tissue of the air-cells, and to increase their size, when not held in check by the pressure of the walls of the thorax upon the lung-bag itself. The lungs are subject, however, to this pressure exerted by the walls of the thorax during the contraction, and to the release of this pressure during the expansion of the thoracic cavity. The pressure that can be exerted by the walls of the thorax on the outside of the lung-bag is much greater than that which results from the atmospheric pressure (air pressure) within the lungs. Therefore, when we wish, as we say, to "take a breath" (inspiration), all we have to do is to reduce the pressure exerted upon the lungs by the chest walls, and to employ those muscular coordinations which increase the intra-thoracic capacity of the lungs (increased chest capacity), thereby causing a partial vacuum in the lung cells of which atmospheric pressure takes advantage, by increasing the size of the cells and thus the amount of air in the lungs. It then follows that if we wish to exhale breath (expiration), we merely have to increase the pressure on the lungs by contracting the walls of the thorax, thereby overcoming the atmospheric pressure exerted within the lungs, and thus forcing the air out of them. It must be remembered that in all these contractions and expansions, the floor of the cavity (diaphragm) plays its part, moving upwards or downwards in sympathy with the particular adjustment of the bony thorax.

Consideration of the foregoing will serve to convince the reader that if anyone desires, either by his own effort or with the help of a teacher, to secure the maximum control and development in breathing, all that he has to do is to be able to command the maximum functioning of the psycho-physical mechanisms concerned with the satisfactory expansion and contraction of the walls of the thoracic (chest) cavity. *It is not necessary for him even to think of taking a breath;* as a matter of fact, it is more or less harmful to do so, when such psycho-physical conditions are present as call for re-education on a general basis.

The crux of the whole matter, then, is how to gain this control in expanding and contracting the chest, as we say, and thus permanently to increase its capacity and mobility. The answer to this question calls for a comprehensive consideration of the primary, secondary and other psycho-physical factors involved.

Naturally, the most potent stimulus to the use of the respiratory mechanisms is the necessity for an adequate supply of oxygen, and for the elimination of carbonic acid gas (poison) from the blood. But we must not overlook the fact that in any attempt to gain for a pupil the desired control and the increased thoracic capacity, the pupil's incorrect use of the mechanisms involved is an impeding factor, and so, in attempts to correct such imperfect use, the first consideration must be to *prevent the psycho-physical activities which are responsible for this defective use* by the development and employment of the pupil's ability to inhibit. This demands from the teacher a correct diagnosis of the pupil's numerous bad habits in connexion with the act of respiration in every-day life, and a comprehensive understanding of the imperfections in sensory appreciation, conception, adjustment and co-ordination which are manifested in these bad habits.

As a result of the diagnosis, the teacher will go on to explain to the pupil why certain readjustments and improved co-ordinations are necessary in his case, and will then give him a reasoned consideration of the *means whereby* these readjustments and improved co-ordinations may be secured. To this end the teacher will first name the preventive guiding orders or directions which the pupil is to give to himself in the way of *inhibiting* the deceptive guiding sensations concerned with the defective use of the mechanisms responsible for what we call bad habits in breathing. The teacher must make certain that the pupil remembers these guiding orders or directions *in the sequence in which they are to be employed.* When this has been done, the pupil may begin the practice in connexion with the work of prevention. This means a series of repeated experiences on the part of the pupil in refusing to try for the "end," and in positively pausing to think of the original faults pointed out by the teacher, and refusing to repeat them.

For instance, suppose that a pupil has a special desire to increase his chest capacity. This desire acts as a stimulus to the psycho-physical processes involved and sets in motion all the unreliable guiding and directing sensations associated with his established idea of chest expansion. The only way, then, by which he can *prevent* the old subconscious habits from gaining the upper hand is for him to *refuse to act* upon this idea. This means that as soon as the idea or desire comes to him *he definitely stops* and says to himself: "No. I won't do what I should like to do to increase my chest capacity, because, if I do what I feel will increase it, I shall only use my mechanisms as I have used them before, and what is the good of that? I know I have been using them incorrectly up to now, else why do I need these lessons?" In other words, he inhibits his desire to act.

The teacher, of course, must decide when the pupil can proceed from the preventive to the next stage of his work. He must then proceed to name for the pupil the new orders in connexion with the satisfactory guiding sensations concerned with the correct use of the mechanisms involved. The pupil should recall and give himself these new guiding orders, whilst the teacher, by means of his manipulation, assists him to secure the correct readjustment and co-ordination (the desired "end"), thus ensuring a series of satisfactory experiences which should be repeated until the bad habits are eradicated and the new and correct experiences replace them and become established.

Repetition of these correct experiences is all that is required to establish a satisfactory use of the co-ordinated psycho-physical mechanisms concerned, when an increase or decrease in the intra-thoracic (chest) capacity can be secured at will, with the minimum of effort and with a mathematical precision. The increase in the intra-thoracic (chest) capacity indicated decreases the pressure on the outside of the lung-bag and causes a momentary partial vacuum in the lungs. This vacuum is promptly filled with air, in consequence of the atmospheric pressure exerted upon the inside of the lung cells, and this process increases the amount of air in the lungs, constituting the act of what we call "taking a breath" (inspiration). The marvellous efficiency of the respiratory machine, when properly employed, becomes apparent when we realize that we have only to continue to employ the same *means whereby* we secure the increase (expansion) to secure the decrease (contraction) of the intra-thoracic capacity, which means that in the process the contracting chest walls exert such increased pressure on the lungs that the air-pressure within is overcome, and the air consequently expelled, this process constituting "expiration"; the expiration and previous inspiration being the completed act of breathing. When a satisfactory, co-ordinated use of the mechanisms concerned with the acts of inspiration and expiration is established, the teacher may then proceed to help the pupil to employ this co-ordinated use in connexion with all vocal effort. This should begin with *whispered* vocalization, preferably the vowel sound "Ah," as this form of vocal use, being so little employed in every-day life, is rarely associated with ordinary bad psycho-physical habits in vocalization.

For this reason, the teacher will begin by helping the pupil to make the expiration on a whispered "Ah." This calls for a knowledge of the psycho-physical "means-whereby" of the use of the organism *in general,* and of the acts of opening the mouth, using the lips, tongue, soft palate, etc., with freedom from stress and strain of the vocal mechanisms, and to this end a definite technique is employed. The process involved prevents sniffing and "sucking in air," undue depression of the larynx and undue stiffening of the muscles of the throat, vocal organs and neck. It also prevents the undue lifting of the front part of the chest during inspiration, its undue depression during expiration, and also many other defects which are developed by any imperfectly co-ordinated person who attempts to learn "breathing" or "deep-breathing," etc., guided by the unreliable sensory appreciation which is always associated with an imperfectly co-ordinated condition of the psycho-physical mechanism.

# PART II
# THE WAY IT WORKS

*Chapter One*

# INHIBITION AS A GOOD WORD

The subconscious self is not a possession peculiar to man, but is in fact more active, in many ways more finely developed, in the animal world. Among some animals the consciousness of danger is so keen that we have attributed it to prescience. The fear of fire in the prairies, of flood, or of the advance of some natural danger threatening the existence of the animal, is evidenced far ahead of any signs perceptible by human senses, and as we cannot, except sentimentally, attribute powers of conscious reasoning to the animal world, it is evident that this "fore-knowledge" is due to a delicate co-ordination of animal senses. Again, we see that animals which have not had their powers dulled by many generations of domestication make the majority of their movements, as we say, "instinctively." They can judge the length of a leap with astonishing accuracy, or take the one certain chance of escape among the many apparent possibilities open to them without an instant's hesitation, and as these powers are evidenced in some cases within a few hours or minutes after the birth of the animal, they are admittedly not the outcome of experience.

The whole argument for the evidence of the possession of a subconscious self by animals can be elaborated to any length, and depends upon facts of observation made over a long period of time. The few examples I have here cited merely illustrate that side of the question which throws into prominence the point of what we may call abnormal powers, or powers which seem to transcend those of human reason so far as it has been developed.

In the second place, however, we are confronted with the unquestionable fact that the subconsciousness can be "educated" below the plane of reason. Acts very frequently performed become so mechanical that they can be repeated without any sense of conscious awareness by the operator. The pianist, after constant rehearsals, will perform the most intricate passage while his attention is engaged with an entirely unrelated subject,—although it is particularly worthy of remark in this connexion, that when such an art as the performance of music falls temporarily into such an automatic repetition, the connoisseur will instantly recognise the loss of some quality—generally spoken of as "feeling"—in the rendering. Again, it appears that in some cases a more or less permanent impression may be made upon the subconsciousness by casual suggestions, often related to fear, even though such suggestions be, in some cases, the result of a single experience. A nervous hysterical subject, already far too willing to submit to the guidance of emotion and what he or she fondly believes to be "instinct" or "intuition" may be so harmfully impressed in this way as to develop any of the many forms of "phobia," which are, as the suffix correctly implies, forms of morbid terror. These are but two instances of the "education" of the subconsciousness below the reasoning plane, but a dozen others will suggest themselves to the reader out of his own experience. The important point is the fact that the phase of being with which we are dealing becomes, as we progress through life, a composite of animal instincts and habits acquired below the plane of reason either by repetition or by suggestion. But before I leave this general conception of the subconsciousness, I must emphasise the fact that up to this point we share the qualities of the subconscious mind with the animal kingdom. For in the lower organisms no less than in that of humanity, this subconsciousness can be educated. The observations of naturalists now confirm the belief that the young of certain birds —the swallow has been particularly instanced—are *taught* to fly by the parent birds; whilst any one who has trained a dog will know how such a trick as "begging" for food may become so habitual as to appear instinctive.

So much for general definition; I come now to the point which marks the differentiation of man from the animal world, and which is first clearly evidenced in the use of the reasoning, intellectual powers of inhibition.

Now it is evident that in the earlier stages of man's development, the inhibition of the subconscious animal powers was frequently a source of danger and of death. Reason, not as yet sufficiently instructed and far-seeing, was an inefficient pilot, and sometimes laid the ship aback when she would have kept before the wind if left to herself. To abandon the metaphor, the control was imperfect, it wavered between two alternatives, and by rejecting the guidance of instinct it suffered, it may be, destruction. But the necessity for conscious control grew as the conditions of life came to differ ever more and more from those of the wild state. This, plainly, was due to many causes, but chiefly to the limitations enforced by the social habit which grew out of the need for co-operation.

This point must be briefly elaborated, for it marks the birth of inhibition in its application to everyday life, and in so doing it demonstrates the growth of the principle of conscious control which, after countless thousands of years, we are but now beginning to appreciate and understand.

It is true that we have evidence of conscious inhibition in a pure state of nature. The wild cat stalking its quarry inhibits the desire to spring prematurely, and controls to a deliberate end its eagerness for the instant gratification of a natural appetite. But in this, and in the many other similar instances, such instinctive acts of inhibition have been developed through long ages of necessity. The domestic kitten of a few weeks old, which has never been dependent on its own efforts for a single meal, will exhibit the same instinct. In animals the inherited power is there; in man also the power is there as a matter of physical inheritance, but with what added possibilities due to the accumulated experience gained from the conscious use of this wonderful force.

The first experience must have come to man very early in his development. As soon as any act was proscribed and punishment meted out for its performance, or as soon as a reward was consciously sought—though its attainment necessitated realised, personal danger—there must have been a deliberate, conscious inhibition of natural desires, which in its turn enforced a similar restraint of muscular, physical functioning. As the needs of society widened, this necessity for the daily, hourly inhibition of natural desires increased to a bewildering extent on the prohibitive side. There grew up first "taboos," then the rough formulation of moral and social law, and on the other hand a desire for larger powers which encouraged qualities of emulation and ambition.

Among the infinite diversity of these influences, natural appetites and the modes of gratifying them were ever more and more held in subjection, and the subconscious self or instinct which initiated every action in the lower animal world fell under the subjection of the conscious, dominating intellect or will. And in this process we must not overlook one fact of supreme importance, viz., man still progressed physically and mentally. It is therefore clear that this control acquired by the conscious mind broke no great law of nature, known or unknown, for, if this acquired control had been in conflict with any of those great, and to us as yet incomprehensible, forces which have ruled the evolution of species, the animal we call man would have become extinct, as did those early saurian types which failed to fulfil the purpose of development and perished before man's first appearance on this earth.

Before we attempt, then, any exact definition of the subconscious self we must have a clearer comprehension of the terms "will," "mind," and "matter," which may or may not be different aspects of one and the same force. More than two thousand years of philosophy have left the metaphysicians still vaguely speculating as to the relations of these three essentials, and personally, I am not very hopeful of any solution from this source. The investigation, though still in its infancy in this form, has taken the shape of an exact science, and it is to that science of psychology as now understood that I look to the elucidation of many difficult problems in the future. Without touching on the uncertain ground of speculative philosophy, I will try, however, to be as definite as may be with regard to my conception of the subconscious self.

In the first place, great prominence has been given to the conception of the subconscious self as an entity within an entity, by the claim made for it that it has absolute control of the bodily functions. This claim depends for its support upon the evidence of hypnotism and of the various forms of auto-suggestion and faith-healing. Under the first heading, we have been told that under the direction of the hypnotist the ordinary functions of the body may be controlled or superseded, as for instance, that a wound may be formed and bleed without mechanically breaking the skin, or that a wound may be healed more rapidly than is consistent with the ordinary course of nature. Under the second heading, which includes all forms of self-suggestion, we have had examples of what is known as stigmatisation,[1] or the appearance on the bodies of hysterical and obsessed subjects of some imitation of the five sacred wounds. Indeed the instances of cures which seem to our uninstructed minds miraculous, and due by inference to the power of faith, are so numerous that no special example need be cited. These and many kindred phenomena have been explained on the hypothesis that the hidden entity when commanded by the will is able to exert an all-powerful influence either beneficent or malignant, the obscure means by which the command may be enforced being variously described. We see at once that the conception of a hidden entity is the primitive explanation which first occurs to the puzzled mind. We find the same tendency in the many curious superstitions of the savage who turns every bird, beast, stone, and tree into a Totem, and endows them with powers of evil or of good, and discovers a "hidden entity" all of a piece with this conception of the subconscious self, in a piece of wood that he has cut from a tree, or a lump of clay that he has modelled into the rude shape of man, bird, or beast.

My own conception is rather of the unity than the diversity of life. And since any attempt to define the term Life would be presumptuous, the definition being beyond the scope of man's present ability, I will merely say that life in this connexion must be read in the widest application conceivable. And it appears to me that all we know of the evolution or development of life goes to show that it has progressed, and will continue to progress, in the direction of self-consciousness. If we grant the unity of life and the tendency of its evolution, it follows that all the manifestations of what we have called the "subconscious self" are functions of the vital essence of life-force, and that these functions are passing from automatic or unconscious to reasoning or conscious control. This conception does not necessarily imply any distinction between the thing controlled and the control itself. This may be inferred from the use of the word "self-conscious," but the further elucidation of this side of the theory is not germane to the present argument.

Now I am quite prepared to accept as facts phenomena of the kind I have instanced, such as unusual cures effected by hypnotism,

[1] There is much evidence on this point, some of it conflicting, but the main fact must be considered above question.

and by the somewhat allied methods of the various forms of faith healing, but I do deny, and most emphatically deny, that either procedure is in any way necessary to produce the same or even more unusual phenomena. In other words, I maintain that man may in time obtain complete conscious control of every function of the body without, as is implied by the word "conscious," going into any trance induced by hypnotic means, and without any paraphernalia of making reiterated assertions or statements of belief.

Apart from my practical experience of the harm that so often results from hypnotic and suggestive treatment, an experience sufficient to demonstrate the dangers of applying these methods to a large majority of cases, I found my objection to these practices on a broad and, I believe, incontrovertible basis. This is that the obtaining of trance is a prostitution and degradation of the objective mind, that it ignores and debases the chief curative agent, the apprehension of the patient's conscious mind, and that it is in direct contradiction to the governing principle of evolution, the great law of self-preservation by which the instinct of animals has been trained, as it were, to meet and overcome the imminent dangers of everyday existence. In man this desire for life is an influence in therapeutics so strong that I can hardly exaggerate its potentiality, and it is, moreover, an influence that can be readily awakened and developed. The will to live has in one experience of mine lifted a woman almost from the grave, a woman who had been operated upon and practically abandoned as dead by her surgeons. A passing thought flashing across a brain that had all but abandoned the struggle for existence, a sudden consciousness that her children might not be well cared for if she died, was sufficient to reawaken the desire for life, and to revivify a body which no medical skill could have saved. But there is no need to quote instances. The fact is recognized, yet how small is the attempt made to use and control so potent a force! The same argument may be also applied to the prostration of the mind as a factor in the popular rest cures which really seek to put the mind, the great regenerating force, out of action.

Returning to my definition of the subconscious self, it will be seen that I regard it as a manifestation of the partly-conscious vital essence, functioning at times very vividly but on the whole incompletely, and from this it follows that our endeavours should be directed to perfecting the self-consciousness of this vital essence. The perfect attainment of this object in every individual would imply a mental and physical ability and a complete immunity from disease that are still dreams of the future. But once the road is pointed, we must forsake the many bypaths, however fascinating, bypaths which lead at last to an *impasse* and necessitate a return in our own footsteps. Instead of this, we must devote our energies along the indicated road, a road that presents, it is true, many difficulties, and is not straight and easy to traverse, but a road that nevertheless leads to an ideal of mental and physical completeness almost beyond our imaginings.

.　　　　.　　　　.　　　　.　　　　.

There has just come to my knowledge an interesting objection to the importance which I attach to the process of inhibition as a primary and fundamental factor in the technique of the scheme I advocate, and the objection is made on the ground that this use of inhibition will cause harmful suppression in the individual concerned. I shall proceed to shew that such an objection is the outcome of a total misunderstanding of the fundamental psycho-physical processes concerned with the application of the preventive principles employed in my technique.

There has been and still is a growing tendency to attempt to free children from undue external restraint, both at home and at school, with the idea of preventing those harmful suppressions supposed to be the result of the inhibitions associated with the imposition of the restraint characteristic of less modern methods. The idea concerned is conceived on a specific and curative basis and is generally accepted, particularly in schools where an effort is being made to create conditions of environment and occupation to meet the pupil's needs. The points I wish to emphasize in this connexion are (1) that the process of inhibition involved is employed in connexion with ideas directly associated with the gaining of "ends," these ideas being the response to a stimulus (or stimuli) arising from some primary desire or need, and (2)—and this is all-important—that the stimulus (or stimuli) to inhibit this response comes from without, and the process of inhibition is *forced* upon the pupil. This means that his desire is thwarted in consequence of compliance with a command from an outside authority, and this could account for the disturbed emotional conditions associated with what is known as suppression.

Now the inhibitory process involved in my technique has little in common with that to which reference has just been made. For the idea concerned with inhibition in my technique is conceived on a general and preventive basis, and the process of inhibition involved is employed primarily in connexion with ideas which are dissociated from any direct attempt to gain an "end," but associated instead with that indirect procedure inseparable from the practical application of the principles concerned with the *means whereby* an end may be gained. These ideas are the response to a stimulus (or stimuli) arising from a reasoned, constructive conscious understanding and acceptance by the pupil of the principles concerned with the *means-whereby,* and as the procedure concerned with the application of these principles involves the prevention of "end-gaining" acts, the performance of which is associated with misdirected activities, it follows that the pupil's acceptance of the need for and efficacy of such procedure includes also his acceptance of the principle of inhibition of primary desires concerned with such "end-gaining" acts. This, again, really means that in the application of my technique the process of inhibition, that is, *the act of refusing to respond* to the primary desire to gain an "end" *becomes the act of responding* (volitionary act) to the conscious reasoned desire to employ the *means whereby* that "end" may be gained.

The stimulus to inhibit, therefore, in this case comes from within, and the process of inhibition is not forced upon the pupil. This means that the pupil's desire or desires will be satisfied, not thwarted, and that there will be present desirable emotional and other psycho-physical conditions which do not make for what is known as suppression in any form.[1]

The tendency of people on a subconscious plane to speak and act without adequate thought or consideration is a particularly marked manifestation, when there is present an unusually potent stimulus to those processes concerned with what are known as

[1] There are many persons who pride themselves on self-control who are really victims of enslavement to a fixed "end," that is, they do not control themselves by stopping to think out the "means-whereby" to their "ends," but by excluding everything which does not agree with the "ends" which they have set up as right and proper. They themselves may contend that their control is purely self-imposed and

prejudice and emotional disturbances. We are all familiar with the phrases, "Why don't you think before you act?", "Think before you speak," and so on. When the human creature's activities are on a plane of constructive, conscious control, he will have reached a standard of development and use of the processes of inhibition (as outlined in the technique which I advocate), which will enable him to apply in practice to his activities in the outside world the very principles concerned with the processes of inhibition which he has applied to the use of his psycho-physical self, with accruing benefit in both spheres of application.

In this connexion I will now give an incident which I think is of particular interest and pertinence as shewing the application of the technique employed in the work of re-education on a general basis to the practical ways of life, and also the analogy which exists between the process of "linking-up" (association of ideas) during the lessons, and the process of linking up what has been gained during those lessons with the experience of every-day life. I also give it in proof of the fundamental value of the principle of inhibition involved.

A pupil of mine, an author, had been in a serious state of health for some time, and had at last reached the point where he was unable to carry on his literary work. After finishing his latest book he passed through a crisis which was described as a "breakdown," with the result that even a few hours of work caused him great fatigue and brought on a state of painful depression. From the outset of his lessons, therefore, I expressly stipulated that he should *stop* and make a break at the end of each half-hour's writing, and should then either do fifteen minutes' work in respiratory re-education, or take a walk in the open air before resuming his writing.

One afternoon he came to his lesson unusually depressed and enervated, and, in response to my enquiries, he admitted that he had been indulging in his literary work that morning from nine till one without a break, in spite of my express stipulation that he must make frequent breaks. I pointed out to him that if he had been

---

not externally imposed, but to other persons it manifests itself as a form of rigidity. On the other hand, control which results from stopping to reason out the *means whereby* desired ends may be secured is unassociated with that rigidity which is inseparable from enslavement to pre-conceived and unreasoned ideas and beliefs, or to hard and fast rules in regard to what is right and proper in conduct and procedure.

continuing his work for four hours without a break, we could not be surprised at the unfortunate result, for, as I explained to him, during deep thought, as in sleep, the activity of the respiratory processes is reduced to a minimum, a very harmful minimum in his case, owing to the inadequacy of his intra-thoracic capacity, this latter condition being one of the symptoms of his breakdown. "But I am unable to stop when once I get into my work," said my pupil. I suggested that if this were so, it must come from some lack of control on his part. "But surely," my pupil objected, "it must be a mistake to break a train of thought?" I answered that my experience went to shew that this was not the case, that, on the contrary, as far as I could see, it should be as easy to break off a piece of work requiring thought, and take it up again, as it is to carry on a train of thought, whilst taking a walk with all its attendant interruptions, and that this should be possible not only without loss of connexion, but with accruing benefit to the individual concerned.

In all this I was really preparing the way to a special end, namely, the attempt to shew my pupil the analogy that existed between the point in question and his difficulty in accomplishing certain simple parts of the technique in his lessons through his disinclination to stop. I wished to convince him that the gaining of control in the simple psycho-physical evolutions in which we were engaged during the lessons meant sooner or later the gaining of control in the practical spheres of his daily life. My pupil had failed to make this all-important connexion between his work in re-education and his outside activities, and therefore the connexion between the difficulty he experienced in "stopping" in his lessons and "stopping" in the midst of his literary work had completely escaped him.

In this, however, he was only in like case with thousands of other well-educated and intelligent people who, in dealing with a situation, fail to make an obvious association of ideas, and so miss most important connecting links between different factors in a case. In this particular instance, had my pupil made the necessary connexion between the difficulty he had in "stopping" in his lessons and "stopping" in his activities outside, this recognition would have given a new meaning, and therefore an added stimulus to the psycho-physical effort upon which the successful working-out of the technique depends.

## Chapter Two

# HOW WE GOT THIS WAY

"Our contemporaries of this and the rising generation appear to be hardly aware that we are witnessing the last act of a long drama, a tragedy and comedy in one, which is being silently played, with no fanfare of trumpets or roll of drums, before our eyes on the stage of history. Whatever becomes of the savages, the curtain must soon descend on savagery forever."—J. G. FRAZER.

The long process of evolution still moves quietly to its unknown accomplishment. Struggle and starvation, the hard fight for existence working with fine impartiality, remorselessly eliminate the weak and defective. New variations are developed and old types no further adaptable become extinct, and thus life fighting for life improves towards a sublimation we cannot foresee. But at some period of the world's history an offshoot of a dominant type began to develop new powers that were destined to change the face of the world.

Speculations as to what first influenced that strange and wonderful development do not come within the province of this treatise, but I should like in passing to point out that the theory and practice of my system are influenced by no particular religion nor school of philosophy, but in one sense may be said to embrace them all. For whatever name we give to the Great Origin of the Universe, in the words of a friend of mine, "we can all of us agree . . . that we mean the same thing, namely, that high power within the soul of man which enables him to will or to act or to speak, not loosely or wildly, but in subjection to an all-wise and invisible Authority." The name that we give to that Authority will in no way affect the principles which I am about to state. In subscribing to them the mechanist may still retain his belief in a theory of chemical reactions no less than the Christian his faith in a Great Redeemer. But through whatever influence these new powers in man came into being I maintain that they held strange potentialities, and, among others, that which now immediately concerns us, the potentiality to counteract the force of evolution itself.

61

This is, indeed, at once the greatest triumph of our intellectual growth and also the self-constituted danger which threatens us from within. Man has arisen above nature, he has bent circumstance to his will, and striven against the mighty force of evolution. He has pried into the great workshop and interfered with the machinery, endeavouring to become master of its action and to control the workings of its component parts. But the machine has as yet proved too intricate for his complete comprehension. He has learned gradually the uses of a few parts which he is able to operate, but they are only a small fraction of the whole.

What then is man's position to-day, and what is his danger? His position is this. In emerging from the contest with nature he has ceased to be a natural animal. He has evolved curious powers of discrimination, of choice, and of construction. He has changed his environment, his food, and his whole manner of living. He has enquired into the laws which govern heredity and into the causes of disease. But his knowledge is still limited and his emergence incomplete. The power of the force we know as evolution still holds him in chains, though he has loosened his bonds and may at last free himself entirely. Thus we come to man's danger.

Evolution—a term we use here and elsewhere in this connection as that which is best understood to indicate the whole operation of natural selection and all that it connotes—has two clearly defined functions; by one of these it develops, by the other it destroys. By an infinitely slow action it has developed such wonders as the human eye or hand; by a process somewhat less tedious it allows any organ that has become useless to perish, such as the pineal eye or (in process) the vermiform appendix, and, if we can estimate the future course, the teeth and hair.

By the change he has effected in his mode of life, man is no longer necessarily dependent upon his physical organism for the means of his subsistence, and in cases where he is still so dependent, such as those of the agriculturist, the artisan, and others who earn a living by manual labor, he employs his muscles in new ways, in mechanical repetitions of the same act, or in modes of labour which are far removed from those called forth by primitive conditions. In some ways the physical type which represents the rural labouring population is, in my opinion, even more degenerate than the type we find in cities, and mentally there can be no comparison between the two. The truth is that man, whether living in town or country, has changed his habitat and with it his habits, and in so doing has involved himself in a new danger, for though evolution may be cruel in its methods, it is the cruelty of a discipline without which our bodies become relaxed, our muscles atrophied, and our functions put out of gear.

The antagonism of conscious as opposed to natural selection[1] has now been in existence for many thousands of years, but it is only within the last century or less that the effect upon man's constitution has become so marked that the danger of deterioration or decay has been thrust upon the attention, not only of scientific observers, but of the average, intelligent individual. No examination of history is necessary in this place to set out a reason for this comparatively sudden realization of physical unfitness. Briefly, the civilization of the past hundred years has been unlike the many that have preceded it, in that it has not been confined to any single nation or empire. In the past history of the world an intellectual civilization such as that of Egypt, of Persia, of Greece, or of Rome, perished from internal causes, of which the chief was a certain moral and physical deterioration which rendered the nation unequal to a struggle with younger, more vigorous and—this is important—wilder, more natural peoples. Thus we have good cause for believing that the danger we have indicated, though as yet incipient only, was a determining cause in the downfall of past civilizations. But we must not overlook the fact that destructive wars and devastating plagues held sway in the earlier history of mankind, and whilst the latter acted as an instrument of evolution in destroying the unfit, the former, by decreasing the population, threw a burden of initiative and energy on the remnant, necessitating the use of active physical qualities in the business of all kinds of production.

[1] It should, however, be clearly understood in this connection that certain laws of natural selection must, so far as we can see, always hold good; and it would not be advisable to alter them even if it were possible. For example, that curious law may be cited which ordains the attraction of opposites in mating and so maintains nature's average. The attraction which a certain type of woman has for a certain type of man, and vice versa is, in my opinion, a fundamental law, and any attempt to regulate it would be harmful to the race. This, however, is no argument against the regulation or prevention of marriages between the physically and mentally unfit.

Now the conditions have altered. Greater scientific attainments in every direction than have ever been known have combated, and will probably in the future overcome the devastating diseases which have decimated the populations of cities, whilst a higher ethical ideal constantly tends to oppose the horrible and repugnant barbarism of war which, with the spread of civilization even to the peoples of the Orient, becomes to our senses more and more fratricidal, a fight of brother against brother.

A hundred years ago Malthus, a prophet if not a seer, recognized our danger and within the past quarter of a century a dozen theorists have proposed remedies less stringent than those advocated by Malthus, but almost equally futile. Among the theorists are those perhaps unconscious reactionaries who advocate the simple life, by a return to natural food and conditions, in endlessly varying ways. To them in their search for natural foods and conditions we would point out that countless generations separate us from primitive man, a lapse of time during which our functions have become gradually adapted to new habits and environment, and that if it were possible by universal agreement for the peoples of Europe to return instantly to primitive methods of living, the effect would be no less disastrous than the reversal of the process, the sudden thrusting of our civilization upon savage tribes whereby, to quote one or two recent examples only, the aborigines of North America, New Zealand, and Japan (the Ainu tribes) have become, or are rapidly becoming, extinct.

When therefore we point out man's power of adaptability in this connexion, the emphasis is thrown on the slowness with which that adaptability is passed on to our descendants and on the relative permanence of the new powers acquired. For our purpose the argument remains good whether we admit or deny the inheritability of acquired characteristics, our point being that in either case the process is necessarily a slow one, though it is plainly more rapid if the hypothesis be true.

From the savage to the civilised state, man passed, as I say, so slowly that the passing in the early stages caused neither difficulties nor changes sufficiently marked to force themselves on our recognition. In other words, the subject of these changes was unconscious of them, and the habit of depending upon these sensory appreciations ("feeling tones," or "sense of feeling") dominant by right in the savage or subconsciously directed state, remained firmly established in the civilized experiences, so that to-day man walks, talks, sits, stands, performs in fact the innumerable mechanical parts of daily life without giving a thought to the psychical and physical processes involved.

It is not surprising that the results have proved unsatisfactory. The evils of a personal bad habit do not reveal themselves in a day or in a week, perhaps not in a year, a remark that is also true of the benefits of a good habit. The effects of the racial habits I am now describing have gone on unnoticed for untold centuries. But in the last hundred years the evil has become so marked that its effect has at last forced itself upon our attention. The failure of subconscious guidance in modern civilization is now being widely admitted, and the consideration of this fact has led a few to the logical conclusion that conscious guidance and control are the one method of adapting ourselves not only to present conditions but to any possible conditions that may arise. We have passed beyond the animal stage in evolution and can never return to it.

For these reasons it becomes necessary, if we would be consistent, to reject at once all propositions for improving our future well-being which can by any possibility be described as reactionary. Even in this brief résumé of man's history one tendency stands out clearly enough, the tendency to advance. When that first offshoot from a dominant type began to develop new powers of intellect, a form was initiated which must either progress or perish. Atavism must be counteracted by the powers of the mind, and reaction is a form of atavism. No return to earlier conditions can increase our knowledge of the secret springs of life, or aid our formulation of world-laws by the understanding of which we may hope to control the future course of development.

The physical, mental, and spiritual potentialities of the human being are greater than we have ever realized, greater, perhaps, than the human mind in its present evolutionary stage is capable of realizing. And the present world crisis surely furnishes us with sufficient evidence that the familiar processes we call civilization and education are not, alone, such as will enable us to come into that supreme inheritance which is the complete control of our own potentialities. One of the most startling fallacies of human thought has been the attempt to inaugurate rapid and far-reaching reforms in the religious, moral, social, political, educational, and industrial spheres of human activity, whilst the individuals by whose aid these reforms can be made practical and effective, have remained dependent upon subconscious guidance with all that it connotes. Such attempts have always been made by men or women who were almost completely ignorant of the one fundamental principle which would so have raised the standard of evolution, that the people upon whom they sought to impose these reforms might have passed from one stage of development to another without risk of losing their mental, spiritual, or physical balance.

For in the mind of man lies the secret of his ability to resist, to conquer and finally to govern the circumstances of his life, and only by the discovery of that secret will he ever be able to realize completely the perfect condition of *mens sana in corpore sano.*

I will now endeavor to put before the reader certain facts concerning stages in the evolution of the human creature, when psycho-physical conditions became present which made for the gradual deterioration of sensory appreciation, indicating possible causes of this deterioration in our sense of feeling and in all our other senses. I shall confine this consideration of man's development to three stages:

(1) the stage when he was guided chiefly by sensory appreciation;

(2) the stage when he was developing the ability to inhibit in specific spheres, and was still, as we say, "physically fit";

(3) the stage when he had still further developed this inhibitory power in specific spheres, but had recognized a lower standard of "physical" fitness which called for a remedy.

Stage 1 (Uncivilized Stage): We are well aware of the higher standard of sensory appreciation (associated with all the sensory experiences involved in the general psycho-physical activities essential to a healthy existence) in the uncivilized as compared with the civilized state. In the stage we are considering the satisfactory condition of the savage creature was maintained by the constant use of the mechanisms in the limited spheres of activity concerned with procuring food, drink and shelter, and with preservation of life from human and other enemies. Under such conditions, and at this stage of evolution, subconscious guidance satisfactorily met his immediate needs. He was unaware, that is, of the *means whereby* he employed his mechanisms in the simplest of every-day activities, and this un-awareness did not matter at this stage.

The reason for this is not far to seek. It is that, at this early period, the standard of co-ordination and of the accompanying sensory appreciation in both sexes was comparatively high, and the needs of uncivilized existence did not call for the continual adapta-tion to rapid changes which civilized life demands.

In fact, the physical co-ordination and development of the savage, like that of the animal which he encountered daily, had reached at that period a fine state of excellence. For if we are justified in believing that the two-footed upright creature inherited from its predecessor on four feet a well-developed and healthy organism (and surely there can be little doubt upon this point), we may assume that it reached the human stage in a condition of health which may be described as relatively high.[1]

Since then, during a slow growth of thousands of years, this human creature had been surely and gradually building up a use and development on the so-called physical side in an environment in which changes but rarely occurred, and which, when they did occur, were comparatively slow, so that his activities would gen-erally consist of the daily repetition of the same series of acts of which the standard of difficulty remained about the same.

But on the so-called mental side his use and development had been comparatively limited in an environment where his chief daily effort would consist of hunting down the animals, birds or fish which constituted his daily food supply, an activity for which his instinct was as sure a guide as that of his prey.

With this relatively high standard of use and development on

---

[1] This does not exclude the possibility of the creature's experiencing occasional aches and pains or even of suffering from specific diseases, but barring such specific troubles, the usual level was a normal one. It is significant in this connexion that primitive man always thinks of disease after the analogy of wounds from arrows, stone bruises, etc., that is, as coming in specifically from without, and the technique of the medicine man is to drive out the foreign substances that have come in; if he sweats the patient, for instance, it is to expel some foreign substance.

the "physical" side and the associated development of the organism in general, his experience of ill-health must have been correspondingly small, but if he ever incurred an illness or met with an injury, there can be little doubt that he would apply as a remedy some specific herb or root which he would know to possess the curative qualities he needed.[1] This act would be a subconscious reaction to the stimulus resulting from the sense of ill-being, in exactly the same way as the act of seeking his daily food was a subconscious reaction to the stimulus resulting from the sense of hunger, and as long *as he possessed a mechanical organism which worked with mechanical accuracy, instinctive procedure served his purpose.* The "specific" cure in these circumstances was in keeping with sane and natural requirements. For just as the automatic, slowly developing, subconscious process called instinct guided him in his daily life when he was well, so, when he was ill, this same mysterious but limiting process would indicate to him the necessary and specific remedy, through the agency of the only part of his organism which was as yet highly developed, namely, his sensory appreciation, which would mean that, in this case, his senses of taste and smell would be working in co-ordination with his stomach and his digestive processes.[2]

Thus we see that, whether he were well or whether he were ill, the subconscious guidance of instinct was reliable in the practically unchanging routine of his daily life, so that, because of its associa-

---

[1] Thus we see that the habit of "taking something" for an ill had a very early origin. This habit led naturally to the coming of the medicine-man. For one of the first channels into which man would direct his developing intelligence would be the discovery of the means of remedying or allaying his physical ills or discomforts. This was bound, sooner or later, to produce men and women who would devote themselves exclusively to the study of such remedies and of the human ills for which the remedies were needed.

[2] Incidentally, it is interesting here to draw attention to the fact that up to this day the majority of people under similar conditions are dominated more or less by their sensory appreciation, and the practical proof that this sensory appreciation has deteriorated lies in the difficulty, known only too well to workers in the curative sphere, of persuading the patient to give up some particular food or drink which he himself knows has caused and is still causing his illness. The same thing holds good in cases where a doctor recommends some food or drink which he knows will be most beneficial to his patient, but is not pleasing to the patient's sense of taste. In nine cases out of ten, the doctor's advice will be ignored, and even where it is followed, it will probably be only because he has brought considerable pressure to bear upon his patient. This means that the patient will have allowed his reasoning processes to be dominated by his deteriorated sensory appreciation.

tion with a reliable sensory appreciation, man would have no need of recourse to the higher directive processes.

Stage II (Early Civilizing Stage): As time went on, reasoning came more and more to illumine the creature's dull and limited existence shewn by the fact that he began to construct rude weapons and to build primitive shelters. This reasoning process was destined to grow and develop through the myriad operations of evolutionary building involved in the new and divers experiences concerned with his progress towards a higher plane. With every advance and with every change which he made in his environment, he began to put into practice a reasoning inhibition which enabled him, within certain well-defined limits, to master or modify for his own purposes the desires and tendencies of that sensory mechanism upon which up to that time he had depended entirely for judgment and direction.

The development and use of this reasoning process marked primitive man's differentiation from the lower animals, but it also marked—and this is even more important from the point of view of man's evolutionary history—the "beginning of the end" of the dominance of instinct as a controlling factor in human activity, so that from this period onwards man could no longer satisfactorily live and move by subconscious guidance alone.

Let us see how his newly awakened processes of reasoning would work in the new sphere. In the early stages of his emergence from the savage state, any changes which took place in his environment would be but slow and gradual, and the consequent demands upon his newly developing, higher directive processes would be correspondingly light. As civilization advanced, however, slowly at first but with increasing rapidity as time went on, man must have been placed more and more in new and untried situations which would inevitably demand from him an increasing use of his reasoning processes. This would be exactly the opposite of what had occurred in the earlier savage state where, as we have seen, conditions had called for a relatively higher development on the so-called physical than on the so-called mental side. It is conceivable, therefore, that the new conditions of civilization would call for a relatively rapid increase in man's use and development on the "mental" as compared with the "physical" side. There can also be little doubt that at this stage he had not become dissatisfied with the results of this changing process, and that he continued to receive from within and without more stimuli to "mental" than to "physical" activities. The further he progressed from the savage state, the more frequent would become such stimuli, and the more urgent the call on him to deal with situations, with the result that he would be forced more and more to develop his reasoning processes, in the constant inhibition of his natural desires to meet the demands of a young and developing society and to make the necessary adjustments to the complex requirements of an advancing civilization.

Man had now arrived at the stage where he had left behind him the environment with which he was familiar and to which his limited experiences had adapted him, and as the pathway of his new experiences inevitably widened out, he was confronted with one of the greatest difficulties experienced in his evolutionary progress on a subconscious basis, namely, that of adapting himself quickly to an environment which continued to change with ever-increasing rapidity, and so continually entailed new psycho-physical experiences.

He did adapt himself, of course, to these new conditions whilst his sensory appreciation was still more or less reliable, else he could not have survived, but it was only in the same way as he had always adapted himself, that is, by trusting blindly to the subconscious guidance of instinct which had served his primitive forefathers in their particular environment. Thus early, it seems, in his civilized career, man presumed subconsciously that he was equipped in every way for any new procedure in life such as sawing, for instance, ploughing, chopping, etc., and even for occupations which, with the progress of time, entailed working more and more in cramped or difficult positions.

We may remember, however, that at this early stage a man had every justification for believing that, if he received either from without or within a stimulus to carry out some new duty, perform some new evolution or adopt some new position in the carrying out of a particular piece of work, he would be able, in all probability, to accomplish his aim with impunity. As far as we can see, nothing as yet had occurred to make him suspect that his sensory appreciation was not reliable or that his standard of coordination was not satisfactory, or that, in adapting his mechanisms to new activities in a *specific* way he might be injuring them in a *general* way, and thus be paving the way for a general deterioration. In all his activities hitherto, such as, for instance, the hunting and fighting of his savage days, he had been accustomed to rely upon the subconscious guidance of his sensory appreciation, and so it was upon this same guidance in the use of himself that he continued to rely for all the new and varied occupations of civilization.

This shews that although he had developed his reasoning processes to some extent in inventing crude weapons, implements, etc., during the early stages of his progress towards the civilized state, he did not apply these reasoning processes to the direction of his psycho-physical mechanisms in the use of himself in the various activities of every-day life. With his reasoning processes thus limited in their use, and with no consciousness as yet of any sense of physical shortcoming, it is most unlikely that man could have received even a slight subconscious hint that his instinct would be in any way affected in the new surroundings and amidst the new experiences of civilization, or that he would ever lose a fraction of that satisfactory "physical" use and development which his race had enjoyed for countless ages, which was then his inheritance, and which he never doubted he was to hand down to his successors for all time.

Had he reasoned the matter out, he would have realized that his instinct was built up from very limited experiences, gained in the uncivilized state where growth was slow and changes rare, so that this instinct could not be expected to meet the demands of a mode of life in which growth was much more rapid and changes more frequent and unforeseen. He would also have realized that many of his instincts were being used less and less in the old way, and consequently were becoming less and less reliable. *It would then have been obvious to him that in order to meet satisfactorily the requirements of his new and changing environment, he must employ new guidance and direction, and that in order to build up this new guidance with the rapidity that his necessities demanded, he must call upon reasoning to supersede instinct (the co-worker of slow development) in the use of his psycho-physical mechanisms. In other words, he would have realized that his primitive psycho-physical equipment must pass from the subconscious to the conscious plane of guidance and direction.*

The centuries passed, bringing with them an increasing scope for the use of man's reasoning processes. Unfortunately, he continued to confine this use of his reasoning processes to the consideration of the relation of "cause and effect," "means and ends" in connexion with his activities in the outside world, both social and physical, and failed to apply this reasoning to the consideration of the relation of "cause and effect," "means and ends" in connexion with the use of his psycho-physical organism. At the same time, the use of his so-called physical mechanisms was being gradually but surely interfered with, partly owing to the change from a standard of daily use to one of comparative inactivity, but chiefly owing to the failure of his instincts to meet the demands made upon them by the activities of the new life.

The results of the failure of man's instincts to meet the new and varied demands of civilization would not manifest themselves at once. For it is reasonable to suppose that as man emerged from the savage state, his instinct was still working satisfactorily and that there was little need for curative measures on account of his comparatively high standard of health. Up till then, the so-called physical self, as being more highly developed, had been the guiding and controlling factor in human activity. It is almost beyond human power to-day to realize that the experiences of millions of years had gone to the building-up of this so-called physical development. The experiences man had gained on the so-called mental side were infinitesimal in comparison.

Henceforward this restless, inquisitive creature, endowed with wonderful potentialities and developing on the so-called mental at a far greater rate than on the so-called physical side, continued to progress in the direction of what we call civilization with ever-increasing rapidity. But his race instincts had not equipped him for such a sudden psycho-physical rush, such a tremendous overbalancing on the so-called mental side, so that he arrived at the new stage breathless, dazed, at a loss, as it were, from the lack of the graduated psycho-physical experiences which had been part and parcel of his earlier growth.[1]

[1] This indicates (1) that conscious, reasoned psycho-physical activity must replace subconscious, unreasoned activity in the processes concerned with making the changes demanded by the ever-changing environment of civilization; (2) that these changes must be made more quickly than heretofore in order to meet this demand

Stage III (Later Civilizing Stage): There came at last a time in the history of man when a number of people became aware of a certain serious shortcoming, and the adoption of "physical exercises" as a remedy is proof that they recognized this shortcoming as a "*physical*" deterioration. This sense of shortcoming and of general lack of well-being was more or less to accompany mankind from that time right on through the different stages of the civilizing process.

I write "was to accompany him" advisedly, because it has done so. I also write that it should not and would not have done so if man had realized that this sense of shortcoming was the signal that he had reached a psychological moment in his career, and that the time had arrived for him to come into his great inheritance, that is, to pass from the subconscious, animal stage of his growth and development to higher and still higher stages of apprehension (conscious reasoning) in connexion with the use of his psycho-physical mechanisms.

Unfortunately, man did not recognize the real significance of this danger signal, for the fact remains that he continued the experiment of guiding himself subconsciously, even though this experiment was already proving a failure, and has since so proved itself, with signs unmistakable which "he who runs may read."

There certainly was some consideration of the position. There was this recognition of a deterioration on the so-called physical side beyond any previously recognized experience of mankind, whilst on the other there may even have been a distinct sense of gain through

---

satisfactorily; and (3) that, with the advance of time, there will be a corresponding call for quickening in this sphere of psycho-physical activity.

In short, the fundamental difficulty arises from the following facts. Uncivilized man depended upon subconscious guidance and control, and probably hundreds of years were occupied in making simple changes, for subconscious activity is very slow in its response to the stimulus of the need of change. Civilized man still depends upon subconscious guidance and control just as he did in the uncivilized state—the tragedy of civilization—but although he has remained satisfied with the form of direction and control by means of which changes have hitherto been made, it would seem that he has become dissatisfied with the time occupied with making changes. It is man's supreme civilizing blunder that he has failed to realize in practice that an adequate quickening of the response to the stimuli, arising from the need for some comparatively rapid change, calls for a corresponding quickening of the spheres of direction and control in the use of the psycho-physical mechanisms involved, such as is possible only on a plane of constructive conscious control.

the increased use and development of the so-called mental processes. But the point I wish to make clear is that, where this unequal development was concerned, there had been an inadequate co-ordinating process at work, a process, in fact, the very opposite of co-ordination and one which has continued, with but few exceptions, in human beings until our own time. Indeed, from its beginnings, the process of civilizing tended to widen the scope for so-called mental and to narrow the scope for so-called physical activities, and, on a basis of subconscious guidance and control, this process meant for the time being a further development on the so-called mental side, but at the cost of an equally distinct if more gradual deterioration on the so-called physical side, with an accompanying deterioration in the standard of sensory appreciation. But it must be remembered that because of the interrelation and interdependence of the mechanisms and potentialities of the organism in the process we call human life, any deterioration on the so-called physical side must, in time, seriously affect the so-called mental side. Enlargement of the spheres of so-called mental activity does not necessarily denote a growth of healthy "mental" activity.[1] This has been proved by man's experiences in civilization up to the moment, a statement borne out by the events of 1914–1919. In fact, the process of civilization has gone hand in hand with a harmful interference with those co-ordinating processes upon which the satisfactory growth of man's psycho-physical organism depends.

This being so, it follows that from the time that man entered the civilized state, human growth on this subconscious basis was bound to be uneven and unbalanced, and this unbalanced development marked the beginning of a new era in human existence. It marked the beginning of an interference with the co-ordinated use of his mechanism as a whole, and particularly with those muscular co-ordinations so essential to his "physical" well-being.

---

[1] "Mental" growth continued even after a deterioration had been recognized in the "physical" self, and this deterioration caused, as it were, one limb of the tree to grow at such a pace that it overbalanced the tree, bent it too much in one direction, seriously disturbing the roots responsible for its equilibrium and healthy growth.

## Chapter Three

# MIND-WANDERING AND
# THOUGHT-GROOVES

The shortcoming to which an individual will awaken will be one which interferes with his immediate activities outside himself, in reading, for instance, or when he is attempting to learn something, or to learn to do something, and, as a matter of fact, the shortcoming that has been recognized as interfering more than any other in this connexion is the shortcoming concerned with his inability, as he would put it, to "keep his mind" on the particular work with which he is immediately engaged; in other words, the shortcoming which is commonly known as "mind-wandering."

Now, what is "mind-wandering?" In the attempt to answer this query, we will begin with a consideration of the psycho-physical processes concerned with direction and control within the human creature in the all-important sphere of self-preservation.

In the beginning of things all growth and development must surely have resulted from a form of consciousness[1] of need. For the growth and development of the creature are and always have been associated with new experiences which involve new activities. These activities—the response to some stimulus or stimuli—result from the consciousness of some need or needs within or without the organism, the presence and recognition of need being essential to the evolutionary process.

The recognition of a need denotes a state of consciousness of a need, and the primary activity (or activities) which is the response to this consciousness of a need or needs involves new experiences in the spheres of direction and control. The process of evolution depends upon the continuous repetition of such primary experiences, this repetition resulting in the establishment of a use (or what is termed habit or instinct) and in the satisfaction of the need or needs.

[1] Many readers may not agree with me on this point, but it will be seen that all that is necessary to my argument is a recognition of the place of need, the requirement of a new way of linking up with environment, so that the rest of my argument is not affected by belief or disbelief on this point.

There can be little doubt that self-preservation (taking the word in its broadest sense) was the most fundamental of the creature's needs, for, first and foremost, the creature itself needed protection and preservation during its attempts to satisfy its specific needs.

This need for self-preservation called for that satisfactory direction and control with which, in this sphere, we find wild animals and savages equipped, inasmuch as, owing to the particular circumstances which obtained in their case, the response to any stimulus arising from a need would be satisfactory in the spheres of direction and control, that is, it would be a response which would enable the creature to employ what would be for him the most satisfactory "means-whereby" to securing the essential "end," self-preservation.

Most of us are aware of the marvellous accuracy in the use of the organism manifested by the wild animal or the savage in the various familiar spheres of activity concerned with self-preservation. The civilized creature does not manifest anything like the same standard of accuracy in the employment of the organism in the spheres of activity concerned with self-preservation. In other words, the civilized human being does not enjoy the same standard of effective direction and control as the savage and the wild animal, and it is the lack of this adequate standard in the human creature which manifests itself as a shortcoming in some sphere of activity, and, as I have said, in the sphere of learning something and learning to do something, the shortcoming most frequently recognized is that known as "mind-wandering."

Now there exists a close connexion between the shortcoming which is recognized as "mind-wandering" and the shortcoming which manifests itself as a seriously weakened response to a stimulus to an act (or acts) of self-preservation. To make this connexion clear, we have only to consider the psycho-physical processes involved in these two shortcomings to realize that in both cases these processes are the same.

For the lack underlying these two shortcomings is the lack of an adequate standard of direction and control in the human creature, manifesting itself, in the one case, in the broad sphere of self-preservation and, in the other, in the specific sphere of learning something or learning to do something.

An act of self-preservation is the response to a stimulus (or stimuli) resulting from a fundamental need, and a satisfactory response depends upon the satisfactory direction and control of the psycho-physical mechanisms which are engaged in the act or acts of self-preservation.

An attempt to learn something or to learn to do something is the natural response to a stimulus (or stimuli) resulting from a wish or need to learn something or to learn to do something, and a satisfactory response depends upon the satisfactory direction and control of the psycho-physical mechanisms which are engaged in the acts of learning or learning to do something.

It will thus be seen that the processes involved in the acts concerned with self-preservation, or with learning or learning to do something, are precisely the same, and it follows that, if in the sphere of self-preservation the direction and control are unsatisfactory, the response to the stimuli concerned with the needs of self-preservation will be unsatisfactory; and, by the same rule, if in the sphere of learning and learning to do, the direction and control are unsatisfactory, the response to the stimuli concerned with the wish or needs in connexion with the acts of attempting to learn something or of learning to do something will likewise be unsatisfactory, and this unsatisfactory response is manifested in every-day life in that shortcoming, so common in our time, called "mind-wandering."

We have now reached the point where we must consider the origin of the conception which led to our giving to this particular manifestation the name of "mind-wandering."

A person decides to learn something or to learn to do something. The conception involved in this decision immediately starts a series of activities of the psycho-physical mechanisms involved, those concerned with direction and control being of vital importance to a satisfactory result, which, in this instance, is the ability to learn something or to learn to do something.

Where a person succeeds in this connexion, he is not likely to become conscious of such a shortcoming as "mind-wandering," for the success of his attempt means that his conception of the act to be performed involves the employment of satisfactory *means whereby* he will be able to gain his desired "end." In such a case, the activities of the psycho-physical mechanisms involved in his attempt will be the result of satisfactory direction and control.

On the other hand, where a person does not succeed in his attempt to learn something or to learn to do something, the failure of his attempt means that there are defects in his conception of the act to be performed, in the sense that this conception does not involve the employment of satisfactory *means whereby* he will be able to gain his desired "end." In such a case, the activities of the psycho-physical mechanisms involved in his attempts will be the result of unsatisfactory direction and control, resulting in a *misdirected* use of the psycho-physical mechanisms, and hence his ability to keep them operating on the satisfactory *means whereby* he will be able to gain his desired "end." The whole procedure is an attempt to communicate with points of vantage along lines of communication which are unreliable, resulting in a shortcoming which reaches the consciousness of the ordinary person as an inability to attend to, or, as we say, to "keep the mind upon" the work in hand; and hence it is called "mind-wandering."

As a matter of fact, the defective use of the mechanisms which is responsible for such conditions cannot be adequately described as "mind-wandering," seeing that it is the manifestation of a harmful and misdirected action and reaction, not only in connexion with those processes commonly spoken of as "mind," but *throughout the whole psycho-physical organism.* It is the manifestation of that imperfectly co-ordinated condition which is associated with an unreliable sense of feeling (sensory appreciation) concerned with unsatisfactory direction and control, and which, in the course of its development, has gradually weakened the response of the human creature to stimuli in the sphere of self-preservation.

In this connexion it is important to remember that the savage creature depended chiefly upon the sense of feeling in the spheres of direction and control, and, as his sense of feeling (sensory appreciation) was comparatively reliable, the activities thus directed and controlled would be associated with an *increasing* response to the stimulus for self-preservation.

The civilized creature also depends chiefly upon the sense of feeling in the spheres of direction and control, but as the sense of feeling (sensory appreciation) in his case has now become harmfully unreliable, the activities thus directed and controlled are becoming more and more associated with a *weakening* response to the stimulus to self-preservation.

This all points to a general weakening in the psycho-physical directing and controlling forces of the human creature,[1] a weakening which has been brought about by the fact that man has continued to depend upon subconscious guidance in his endeavours to meet the demands of the civilizing plan, and to rely upon instincts which have survived their usefulness and upon the harmful guidance of defective sense registers (feeling).

Experience follows experience in the human creature's activities, some of these experiences satisfactory, but the majority unsatisfactory, and the creature may be satisfied for the moment, only to be again dissatisfied, however, with the varying results of attempted accomplishment; and the psycho-physical experiences involved do not make for confidence in regard to any attempts which he may be forced to make in the future to meet the demands of civilization.

When conditions such as these are present in the human creature, success is hardly possible; indeed, failure will be almost certain to result, even though he may devote to the accomplishment of his aims the time deemed necessary to ensure success. The natural result of his experiences of failure or comparative failure is that in time he will come to give consideration to the cause or causes involved in these experiences, and this consideration is of special interest to us, because it practically always leads him to the

---

[1] The fact that an individual happens to exhibit satisfactory specific direction and control in some particular activity does not confute this statement; indeed, only serves to strengthen it.

In this connexion I have found in my professional work that too often a person will consider a psycho-physical experience to be quite satisfactory, when I, as an expert, know it to be in reality unsatisfactory. In such a case, the supposedly satisfactory experience is a delusive and harmful experience, on the part of the person concerned, of feeling and thinking he is right when he is actually wrong. In fact, the experience is really an unsatisfactory one, but he does not know it; and so, when later he becomes dissatisfied, he does not attribute his dissatisfaction to his own psycho-physical experiences, but to other people, surroundings, "something wrong somewhere," always believing the cause to be without instead of within the organism.

same conclusion, namely, that his failure is due to "mind-wandering."

Let us now follow out his consideration of the facts in detail. He sets out to learn something or to learn to do something and proceeds, as he would put it, to "give his mind to" his work, in accordance with his conception of this phrase. But he soon discovers that his "mind" is not "on his work," that it has become more occupied, as it were, with some other trend of thought. He therefore proceeds to make a special effort, as he would say, to "keep his mind on" the original task in hand.

Now it is highly probable that he has never given consideration to the *means-whereby* required for such a special effort, for if he had, he would probably have awakened to the fact that he did not have within his control the *means whereby* a special effort of this kind could prove satisfactory. However this may be, the fact remains that in spite of all his efforts to "keep his mind on" what he is doing, the process he thinks of as "mind-wandering" is repeated, with the result that after a certain number of repetitions of this experience, he becomes convinced that the cause of his failure is his *inability* to "keep his mind on" what he is doing.

Just think of the psycho-physical disaster that is here indicated, for it means that the human creature has reached that dangerous stage in connexion with the employment of his psycho-physical mechanisms when the response to a stimulus arising from a need is ineffective, erratic and produces a state of confusion.

The seriousness of this inability of the human creature to "keep his mind on" what he is doing is widely recognized, and this recognition has led to the almost universal adoption of what is called concentration as the cure for "mind-wandering." Unfortunately, this remedy, as I shall shew later, is in itself a most harmful and delusive psycho-physical manifestation, and has been adopted without any consideration being taken of its effect upon the organism in general or of the psycho-physical processes involved in what is called "learning to concentrate."

We must always remember that the vast majority of human beings live very narrow lives, doing the same thing and thinking the same thoughts day by day, and it is this very fact that makes it so necessary that we should acquire conscious control of the mental and physical powers as a whole, for we otherwise run the risk of losing that versatility which is such an essential factor in their development.

If, at this point, the reader feels inclined to analyse these habits and to set about a control of them, I will give him one word of preliminary advice, "Beware of so-called concentration."

This advice is so pertinent to the whole principle that it is worth while to elaborate it. Ask any one you know to concentrate his mind on a subject—anything will do—a place, a person, or a thing. If your friend is willing to play the game and earnestly endeavours to concentrate his mind, he will probably knit his forehead, tense his muscles, clench his hands, and either close his eyes or stare fixedly at some point in the room. As a result his mind is very fully occupied with this unusual condition of the body which can only be maintained by repeated orders from the objective mind. In short, your friend, though he may not know it, is not using his mind for the consideration of the subject you have given him to concentrate upon, but for the consideration of an unusual bodily condition which he calls "concentration." This is true also of the attitude of *attention* required for children in schools; it dissociates the brain instead of compacting it. Personally, I do not believe in any concentration that calls for effort. It is the wish, the conscious desire to do a thing or think a thing, which results in adequate performance. Could Spencer have written his *First Principles,* or Darwin his *Descent of Man,* if either had been forced to any rigid narrowing effort in order to keep his mind on the subject in hand? I do not deny that some work can be done under conditions which necessitate such an artificially arduous effort, but I do deny that it is ever the best work. Nor will I admit that such a case as that of Sir Walter Scott can logically be argued against this view. For the real earnest wish to write the Waverly novels was there, even if it originated in the desire to pay the debts he took upon himself, and not in the desire to write the novels because he took a pleasure in the actual performance. Briefly, our application of the word "concentration" denotes a conflict which is a morbid condition and a form of illness; singleness of purpose is quite another thing. If you try to straighten your arm and bend it at the same moment, you may exercise considerable muscular effort, but you will achieve no result, and the analogy applies to the endeavour to delimit the powers of the brain by concentration, and at the same time to exercise them to the full extent. The endeavour represents the conflict of the two postulates "I must" and "I can't"; the fight continues indefinitely, with a constant waste of misapplied effort. Once eradicate the mental habit of thinking that this effort is necessary, once postulate and apprehend the meaning of "I wish" instead of those former contradictions, and what was difficult will become easy, and pleasure will be substituted for pain. We must cultivate, in brief, the deliberate habit of taking up every occupation with the whole mind, with a living desire to carry each action through to a successful accomplishment, a desire which necessitates bringing into play every faculty of the attention. By use this power develops, and it soon becomes as simple to alter a morbid taste which may have been a life-long tendency as to alter the smallest of recently acquired bad habits.

The following is an interesting experience with a pupil who was strongly inclined to a belief in the value and power of concentration. The pupil contested vigorously my attacks on the object of her faith, as practised in accordance with the orthodox conception. She put forward the usual arguments, of course, and I quite failed to make any impression on her mental attitude towards the vexed question under discussion. But at last, some days after our first encounter, my opportunity came. We were not at the time directly discussing concentration, but we were dealing with kindred subjects, and presently my pupil began to speak of the attitudes adopted by people towards the things in life that they like or dislike to do. Her own plan, she said, with a touch of pride, had been to develop the habit of keeping her mind on other and more pleasant subjects whenever she had been engaged in a task that was unsympathetic to her, and she had so far succeeded in the cultivation of this habit that the disagreeable sensations of any unpleasant duty were no longer experienced by her. I then put one or two questions to her and elucidated among other facts that for years she had been unable "to concentrate" when reading and that this difficulty was becoming constantly more pronounced. Fortunately this instance opened those locked places of her intelligence that I had been unable to reach by argument. I showed her how she had been cultivating a most harmful mental condition, which made concentration on those duties of life which pleased her appear as a necessity. She had been constructing a secret chamber in her mind, as harmful to her general well-being as an undiagnosed tumor might have been to her physical welfare. I am glad to say that she came to admit the truth of my original position and has since begun her efforts to carry out the suggestions I offered for the correction of her bad habit.

And in all such efforts to apprehend and control mental habits, the first and only real difficulty is to overcome the preliminary inertia of mind in order to combat the subjective habit. The brain becomes used to thinking in a certain way, it works in a groove, and when set in action, slides along the familiar, well-worn path; but when once it is lifted out of the groove, it is astonishing how easily it may be directed. At first it will have a tendency to return to its old manner of working by means of one mechanical unintelligent operation, but the groove soon fills, and although thereafter we may be able to use the old path if we choose, we are no longer bound to it.

# PART III
# WHAT IT IMPLIES

*Chapter One*

# AFTER THE BOMB

The combined efforts of men and women in many parts of the world have resulted in the production of the atomic bomb. This means that they have succeeded in harnessing energy which, when released, can cause devastation on a scale not previously experienced. As a human achievement the atomic bomb is hailed with huzzahs; as a means of destruction it is viewed with horror; as a possible means of the destruction of civilization it is universally feared. Only as a possible aid in supplying future needs of mankind, and thus tending to improve his way of life, is it welcomed by many. But apart from and above all these considerations and possibilities, it will be welcomed by people who now see that the advent of the bomb will force mankind to cry a HALT in many directions, particularly by those people of foresight who have long since realized that it has become essential to cry a universal halt: this, in order that a change can be made in human reactions and in the relations of human beings with each other, based as these are on a way of living that has become unbalanced, and is becoming more so, with increasing rapidity the world over.

Mankind is now faced with new, unexpected, and tremendous problems. An all-important one is that of human relations, for the solution of this problem calls for knowledge of means whereby human reactions can be changed, controlled, and gradually improved. Unfortunately, comparatively few people have ever come into contact with such knowledge. Had this been otherwise, sufficient people might have been so influenced in foresight and outlook by the change that the crisis of 1914–1918, and the rapidly following world crisis of 1939–1945, could have been prevented. But all this, as we shall see, was inevitable when we remember that throughout his long career man has been content to make progress in acquiring control of nature in the outside world, without making like progress in acquiring its essential accompaniment, the knowledge of *how to control nature within himself*—that is to say, how to control his own reactions to the outside world. Up to

87

now he has been so engrossed with the making of changes in the means whereby he could acquire what he considered necessary to his needs in inanimate things, that he has failed to give equal thought to the means whereby he can change and control his animate self. Consequently, as time has gone on, his achievements in controlling nature in the outside world have been discounted by a disintegration within his psycho-physical organism, so that he continually errs in his judgment of relative values and fails in his relations with his fellow-men. Meanwhile he is becoming less and less able to change and control his reactions, even when he attempts to do this by the use of means which he approves and which he tries as best he can to put into practice. The urgency for directing attention to exploring this field of activity is obvious when we consider that, on account of this one-sided development, man has created in the atomic bomb a Frankenstein monster which, if not handled wisely, will prove a constant danger to all, because he has not developed that self-awareness and control of his reactions that is needed if he is to keep control over the monster he has created. As it is, he appears stunned and bewildered by this, his latest discovery, and is afraid to trust himself or his fellow-men with the knowledge that led to its discovery, lest they should react to it in a way that would bring irreparable destruction on the world. There is implied in this a frank admission of the present unsatisfactory nature of man's reaction in general, and this should prove a "blessing in disguise" if he realizes that this nature must be changed and improved if in the future he is to escape the harmful effects which have resulted in the past from his attempts to meet adequately the demands involved in adapting himself to the constant, and progressively more rapid, changes in the world outside of himself. Such a change in the nature of human reaction is essential if mankind is not to remain saddled with frustrating static and obsolete beliefs, ideas, conceptions, and relative values which have long since outlived their usefulness. Obsolete indeed as were many of our ideas, conceptions, beliefs, and so on before the advent of the present crisis, the past few years have completely altered the foundations of our previous ways of life, and it has become a matter of prime necessity to re-examine the pedigree of all such ideas, conceptions, and beliefs with which our overt activities are associated.

To succeed in this, and to set about making the necessary changes to this end, we shall be forced to come to a FULL STOP. This may well prove to be the most difficult and valuable task man has ever undertaken until now, for he has gradually been losing a reliable standard of control of reaction, and the ability to take the long view, in his efforts to improve his conditions when he is faced with the need for changing habits of thought and action. This should not surprise anyone who remembers that in most fields of activity man's craze is for speed and for the short view, because he has become possessed by the non-stop attitude and outlook: he is a confirmed end-gainer, without respect to the nature of the means whereby he attempts to gain his desired end, even when he wishes to employ new means whereby he could change his habits of thought and action.

These habits of reaction which hold him in slavery are the inevitable accompaniments of his out-of-date beliefs and the associated judgments which are too often unsound and frustrating. He will therefore find it difficult to take the long-view outlook of his activities which is inseparable from the ability to STOP when faced with the need for changing habits of thought and action. Man, controlled by impulse and instinct at this stage of his evolution, rarely fails to react according to pattern, no matter in what circumstances. He may claim to be an advocate of freedom *of* thought and action, and may even be a person who acts up to this theory in his daily living; but he cannot, in consequence, claim to be able to put into practice that greatest of all attainments—freedom *in* thought and action—until he has gained that knowledge of the means whereby he can command the best use and functioning of himself in activity, which is essential to change and control of reaction in the basic sense.

By these means, as can be proved by *operational verification,* we are enabled *in process* to bridge the gulf which has for too long separated subconsciousness and consciousness in the control of reaction, and at the same time to widen the gulf between the human and the animal stages of evolution. Full comprehension of the need for the employment of these means could change and improve the basic nature of man's impulsive and instinctive reactions which have developed hand in hand with his static beliefs and outlook. Man's basic nature has not changed as it should have done during past centuries in respect of conscious direction of his use of himself or in regard to his judgment and control in human relations. Hence on every hand he is faced with the impeding effects of "emotional gusts," such as are associated with the too common and frustrating human failings which are manifested in prejudice, jealousy, greed, envy, hatred and the like. These are the outcome of reactions which ruin man's chances of establishing such relations in national and international affairs as could lead to a better understanding of what is essential to the engendering of goodwill and peace in a world in which changing conditions and new discoveries in the outside world make new and ever-increasing demands for increasing change in, and control of, human reaction.

## Chapter Two

# CHILD TRAINING AND EDUCATION

Every child is born into the world with a predisposition to certain habits, and furthermore, the child of to-day is not born with the same development of instinct that was the congenital heritage of its ancestors a hundred or even fifty years ago. Many modern children, for example, are born with recognizable physical disadvantages that are the direct result of the gradually deteriorating respiratory and vital functioning of their forbears.

For many months, the period varying with the sex and ability of the individual, the vital processes and movements are for all practical purposes independent of any conscious control, and the human infant remains in this helpless, dependent condition much longer than any other animal. The habits which the child evidences during this protracted period are those hereditary predispositions which are early developed by circumstance and environment, habits of muscular uses, of vital functioning, and of adaptability. If it were possible to analyze the tendencies of a child when it is, say, twelve months old, we could soon master the science of heredity which is at present so tentative and uncertain in its deductions, but the child's potentialities lie hidden in the mysterious groupings and arrangement of its cells and tissues, hidden beyond the reach of any analysis. The child is our material; within certain wide limits we may mould it to the shape we desire. But even at birth it is differentiated from other children; our limits may be wide but they are fixed. Within those limits, however, our capacity for good and evil is very great.

There are two methods by which a child learns. The first and, in earlier years, the predominant method is by imitation, the second is by precept or directly administered instruction, positive or negative.

With regard to the first method, parents of every class will admit the fact not only that children imitate those who are with them during those early plastic years, but that the child's first efforts to adapt itself to the conditions surrounding it are based almost exclusively on imitation. For despite the many thousand years during which some form of civilization has been in existence, no child has yet been born into the world with hereditary instincts tending to fit it for any particular society. Its language and manners, for instance, are modelled entirely on the speech and habits of those who have charge of it. The child descended from a hundred kings will speak the language and adopt the manners of the East End should it be reared among these associations; and the son of an Australian aboriginal would speak the English tongue and with certain limitations behave as a civilized child if brought up with English people.

No one denies this fact; it has been proved and accepted, yet how often do we seek to make a practical application of our knowledge? Although the science of heredity is still tentative and indeterminate, no reasoning person can doubt from this and other instances that in the vast majority of cases at least, the influence of heredity can be practically eradicated. Personally, I see very clearly from facts of my own observation that when the characteristics of the father and mother are analyzed, and their faults and virtues understood, a proper training of the children will prevent the same faults and encourage the same virtues in their children.

To appreciate to the utmost the effect of training upon the children, we must remember that the first tastes, likes, or dislikes of the infant begin to be developed during the first two or three days after birth. Long before the infant is a month old, habits, tending to become fixed habits, have been developed, and if these habits are not harmful, well and good. The first sense developed is the sense of taste, a sense that develops very quickly and needs the most careful attention. Artificial feeding is in itself a very serious danger, but when this feeding is in the hands of careless or ignorant persons the danger becomes increased a hundredfold. An instance of this is the common idea that considerable quantities of sugar should be added to the milk. This is done very often to induce the child to take food against its natural desire. It may be that the child has been suffering from some slight internal derangement, and Nature's remedy has been to affect the child with a distaste for food in order to give the stomach a rest. Then the unthinking mother tempts the child with sugar, and all sorts of internal trouble may follow. But in such a case as this the taste for a particular thing, such as sugar, is encouraged, and apart from the direct harm which may result, the habit becomes the master of the child, and may rule it through life; the child, in fact, is sent out into the world the slave of the sense of taste.

Unfortunately, in ninety cases out of a hundred, children up to the age of six or seven years are allowed to acquire very decided tastes for things which are harmful. Women are not trained for the sphere of motherhood, they do not give these matters the thought and attention they deserve, and hence they do not understand the most elementary principles concerning the future welfare of their offspring in such matters as feeding and sense guidance. Children are not taught to cultivate a taste for wholesome, nourishing foods, but are tempted, and their incipient habits pandered to, by such additions as the sugar I have more particularly cited.

At the present time I know a child of five years old whose taste is already perverted by the method, or lack of method, I have indicated. This child dislikes milk unless undue quantities of sugar are added, will not eat such food as milk puddings or brown bread, and has a strong distaste for cream. It is almost impossible to make the child eat vegetables of any kind, but he is always ready to take large quantities of meat and sweets. The child is already suffering from malnutrition and serious internal derangement. The latter would be greatly improved by small quantities of olive oil taken daily, but it is only with the greatest difficulty that the child can be induced to take it. If he lives with his parents for the next ten years, he will grow into a weak and ailing boy, and will suffer from the worst forms of digestive trouble and imperfect functioning of the internal organs.

Thus we see that in such instances the mischief begins very early in the life of the child, and it is carried on and exaggerated with every step in its development. Even in babyhood precept and coercion should come into play. Usually when the child cries, little effort is made to discover the cause. Often the child is soothed by being carried up and down the room. It is wonderful how soon the infant begins to associate some rudiments of cause and effect. The child who is unduly pandered to will soon learn to cry whenever it desires to be rocked or dandled, and thus the foundations of pandering to sensation are quickly laid.

But as the child comes to the observant age its habits begin to grow more quickly. We have admitted that a child imitates its parents or nurses in tricks of manner and speech, yet we do not stop to consider that it will also imitate our carriage of the body, our performance of muscular acts, even our very manner of breathing. This faculty for imitation and adaptation is a wonderful force, and one which we have at our command if we would only pause to consider how we may use it in the right way. The vast majority of wrong habits acquired by children result from their imitation of the imperfect models confronting them. But how many parents attempt to put a right model before their children? How many learn to eradicate their own defects of pose and carriage so that they may be better examples to the child? How many in choosing a nurse will take the trouble to select a girl whom they would like their children to imitate? Very, very few, and the reason is simple. In the first place they do not realize the harmful effect of bad example, and, in the second, the great majority of parents have so little perception of truth in this matter that they are incapable of choosing a girl who is a good specimen of humanity, and are sublimely unconscious of their own crookedness and defects.

Children too accept their parents' defects as normal and admirable. The boy of 12 or 14 never dreams for instance that his father's protruding stomach is anything but the condition proper to middle-age, and often, doubtless, figures to himself the time when he will arrive at the same condition. The time will come when such things as these—I refer to the abnormality of the father —will be considered a disgrace. What then can we hope from these parents who are at the present time so unfit, so incapable of teaching their own children the primer of physical life? And I may note here that this principle has a wider application than that of the nursery; it holds, also, in connection with the model of physical well-being set by the teachers in all primary and secondary schools. There is no need for me to elaborate this theme. The iniquity of allowing children to be trained in physical exercises, in our Board Schools for instance, by a teacher who is obviously physically unfit, is sufficiently glaring.

The crux of the whole question is that we are progressing towards conscious control, and have not yet realized all that this progress connotes. Children, as civilization becomes continually more the natural condition, evidence fewer and fewer of their original savage instincts. In early life they are faced by two evils, if they are developed on the subconscious plane. If they are trained under the older methods of education they become more and more dependent upon their instructors; if under the more recent methods of *"free expression"* (to which I shall presently refer at some length) they are left to the vagaries of the imperfect and inadequate directions of subconscious mechanisms that are the inheritance of a gradually deteriorated psycho-physical functioning of the whole organism.

In such conditions it is not possible for the child to command the kinæsthetic guidance and power essential to satisfactory free expression, or indeed to any other satisfactory form of expression for its latent potentialities. As well expect an automobile, if I may use the simile, to express its capacity when its essential parts have been interfered with in such a way as to misdirect or diminish the right impulses of the machinery.

The child of the present day, once it has emerged from its first state of absolute helplessness, and before it has been trained and coerced into certain mental and physical habits, is the most plastic and adaptable of living things. At this stage the complete potentiality of conscious control is present but can only be developed by the eradication of certain hereditary tendencies or predispositions. Unfortunately, the usual procedure is to thrust certain habits upon it without the least consideration of cause and effect, and to insist upon these habits until they have become subconscious and have passed from the region of intellectual guidance.

I will take one instance as an example of this, the point of right-and-left-handedness. We assume from the outset, and the superstition is so old that its source is untraceable, that a child must learn to depend upon its right hand, to the neglect of its left. This superstition has so sunk into our minds by repetition that it has become incorporated in our language. "Dexterous" stands for an admirable, and "sinister" for an inauspicious quality, and we may even find ignorant people at the present day who say that they would never trust a left-handed person. As a result of this attitude and of the absolute rule laid down that a child must learn to write and use its knife with the right hand only, the number of ambidextrous people is limited to the few who, by some initial accident, used their left hand by preference and were afterwards taught to use their right. In a fairly wide experience I do not remember having heard of a father or mother who has said: "This child may become an artist or a pianist," for example, "and may therefore need to develop the sensitiveness and powers of manipulation of the left hand as well as the right," although I have known of many cases where much time and trouble had to be expended in acquiring the uses of the left hand later in life, such cases as those of persons suffering from writer's cramp and dependent for their living on their ability to use a pen.

I have cited this example of right-handedness because it exhibits the pliability of the physical mechanism in early life, and the manner in which we thoughtlessly bind it to some method of working, without ever stopping to think whether that method is good in itself, or whether it is the one adapted for the conditions of life into which the child will grow. We thrust a rigid rule of physical life and mental outlook upon the children. We are not convinced that the rule is the best, or even that it is a good rule. Often we know, or would know if we gave the matter a moment's consideration, that in our own bodies the rule has not worked particularly well, but it is the rule which was taught to us, and we pass it on either by precept, or by holding up our imperfections for imitation and then we wonder what is the cause of the prevailing physical degeneration!

What is intended by these methods of education is to inculcate the accumulated and inferentially correct lessons derived from past experience. It is true that the lesson varies according to the religious, political, and social colour of the parent and teacher, but speaking generally, the intention would be logical enough, if we could make the primary assumption that each generation starts from the same point,—the assumption, in other words, that a baby is born with the same potentialities, the same mental abilities and assuredly the same physical organism whether he be born in the 16th or the 20th century.

And even as recently as a hundred years ago, that assumption might have been made with some show of reason. For the changes were so slight and have evolved so slowly as to attract little attention. Granted similar conditions of parentage and upbringing, the differences between the child of 1800 A. D. and that of 1700 A. D. were hardly noticeable.

That statement, however, does not apply to the child of today. For many years past there have been unrest and dissatisfaction in the world of education. New methods have been tried, superimposed for the most part on the top of the older ones, and even more daring experiments have been made, experiments which sought to throw over the old traditions, bag and baggage. All these trials have so far failed, in my opinion; and one reason for the failure has been due to the fact that educationalists as a body have been unable to recognize the obvious truth that the child of the twentieth century cannot be judged by the old standards.

This truth is so evident to me that I hesitate at the necessity to prove it. It seems incredible to me that any one of my generation could fail to realize the extraordinary differences between the contemporaries of his own growth and the children of our present civilisation. I could produce a dozen instances of this difference, but one must suffice in this place. It is, however, an example that is peculiarly typical. For I remember, and my experience has not been in any way an abnormal one, the facility with which the children of my generation learnt the uses of common tools. In a sense they may be said to have inherited a certain dexterity in the handling of such things as a hammer, knife, or saw. Today many parents are greatly impressed if a child of from 2½ to 6 years old can use one of these implements with a reasonable show of efficiency. I have known fathers and mothers representative of the average parent of today who find any instance of this efficiency in their own children an almost startling thing and certainly matter for boast to their relations and friends.

Unhappily the real difference goes far deeper than this superficial effect would at first seem to indicate. The early attempts of the modern child to employ his physical endowment in such common and necessary acts as walking, running, sitting or speaking, are far below the standard of ability that I remember a generation ago. The standard of kinæsthetic potentiality has been lowered. Elements that I will not attempt to trace, lest I be tempted on to the fascinating ground of evolutionary theory, have intervened most amazingly in the past thirty years, and the most evident result of this intervention has been the marked change in the subconscious efficiency of the modern child.

Thus, even from the birth of the infant, our problem is not precisely that of the old educationalists; and this primary congenital difference between the children of two generations has been, and is being, exaggerated in the nurseries of the independent classes both in England and America. (Doubtless in other countries of Europe the same effects are being produced, but I prefer to speak only of that which I have observed and closely studied for myself.) There is still a tendency to take all responsibility and initiative away from the child of wealthy parents. Nurses first and governesses later perform every possible act of service that shall relieve the child of trouble. It is not even allowed to invent its own games. Toys are supplied in endless quantities, expensive, ingenious toys, that need no imaginative act to transform them into reduced models of the motors, trains, or animals they are manufactured to represent, and some one, some adult, is always at hand to amuse the child and *teach him how to play.* I must italicise the absurdity of that last sentence. For what does this teaching mean, if it does not mean that it is seeking to substitute the adult idea of play for the childish one? In my day, any old brick played the part of a train or a horse, and in the mental act required to see the reality under so uncompromising a guise my imagination was exercised.

But although a petrifying method of teaching and supervision is still practised, the reaction against it has already set in both in England and America. Unhappily that reaction has been too violent as such reactions commonly are. From one extreme of permitting the child no opportunity of the exercise of independent thought and action, we have flown to the other in adopting the principle which is now known as "Free Expression"—a principle which I can show to be no less harmful than over-supervision. In fact so far as the physical expression of a child is concerned, the methods of Free Expression are even more dangerous than those of the opposite school.

In England, this movement towards "Free Expression" has not so far been crystallized into a definite propaganda, nevertheless a number of thoughtful but unhappily inexpert parents are trying to adopt the principle in their own homes. Mr. Shaw's Preface to his *Misalliance* puts the theory of the method in a very clear and convincing argument. His main assumption is as follows: "What is a child? An experiment. A fresh attempt to produce the first man made perfect; that is, to make humanity divine. And you will vitiate the experiment if you make the slightest attempt to abort it into some fancy figure of our own. . . ." That represents, of course, an idealist attitude, and every idealistically minded parent in Great Britain who reads that Preface of Mr. Shaw's on "Parents and Children" at once attempts to put the theory into practice. The results, if the theory is persisted in, will be disastrous; and although in many cases the parents realize their error by practical experience before the child reaches the age of seven or so, certain cases I have seen demonstrate all too clearly that much mischief is being done even at the age of seven; faults and bad habits have become so far established that it is sometimes very hard to eradicate them.

And in America the mischief is going further still. So called "free" schools have been instituted which, although they may differ in the detail of their methods, are based on the same underlying principles. As far as I have examined the theory and practice of these schools their purposes are:

(1) To free the child as far as possible from outside interference and restraint.
(2) To place him in the right environment and then to give him materials and allow him activities through which he may "freely express himself."

Now this presupposes, firstly, that the child if left to himself has the power of expressing himself adequately and freely; secondly, that through this expression, he can educate himself. How far both these suppositions are fallacies will be understood by any one who has followed my argument and my citations of actual cases even up to this point; but the matter is so important that I do not hesitate to bring forward further evidence to establish my objection to this new and dangerous method.

I will begin by drawing attention to the practical side of two of the channels for self-expression, which are specially insisted upon in schools where the new mode is being practised, namely, dancing and drawing. A friend of mine always refers to them as the two D's, a phrase that refers very explicitly to these two forms of damnation when employed as fundamentals in education.

The method of the "Free Expressionists" is to associate music with the first of these arts. Now music and dancing are, as every one knows, excitements which make a stronger emotional appeal to the primitive than to the more highly evolved races. No drunken man in our civilization ever reaches the stage of anæsthesia and complete loss of self-control attained by the savage under the influence of these two stimuli. But in the schools where I have witnessed children's performances, I have seen the first beginnings of that madness which is the savage's ecstasy. Music in this connection is an artificial stimulus and a very potent one. And though artificial stimuli may be permissible in certain forms of pleasure sought by the reasoning, trained adult, they are uncommonly dangerous incitements to use in the education of a child of six.

Full-grown men and women will admit that they can become "drunk" with music and by "drunk" I mean that the motions of the subconsciousness are excited to such a pitch that they take control, until they completely dominate the reasoning faculties. Alcohol produces this result by partial paralysis of the peripheral cilia, music and dancing by overrelaxation of the whole kinæsthetic system. In the latter case, however, no evil effects can be produced in the first instance, without the reasoning consent or submission of the subject. Savages and *young children have not yet learnt to withhold that consent.*

And altogether apart from this question of intoxication—to which by the way every individual is not susceptible—these unrestrained, unguided efforts of the children to dance are likely to prove extremely harmful. I have watched while first one air and then another has been played on the piano, the intention of these changes being to convey a different form of stimulus with each air, and I admit that the children responded in accordance with the more or less limited kinæsthetic powers at their command. But it was very obvious to me that all these little dancers were more or less imperfectly co-ordinated; that the idea projected from the ideomotor centre constantly missed its proper direction; that subconscious efforts were being made that caused little necks to take up the work that should have been done by little backs; that the larynx was being harmfully depressed in the efforts to breathe adequately causing both inspiration and expiration to be made through the open mouth instead of through the nostrils; and that the young and still pliable spines were being gradually curved backwards and the stature shortened when the very opposite condition was essential even to a satisfying æsthetic result.

And when we realise that the teachers who witness these lessons are entirely ignorant of the ideal physical conditions that are proper to children, and so are wofully unaware of the dangerous defects that are being initiated by these efforts to dance, we must admit that, as practised, this particular form of free expression is being encouraged at a cost that far outweighs any imagined advantage.

The second ominous "D" is drawing, and this comes into another category of damnation, since mental rather than physical effects are concerned, although the latter are involved both in the harmful, uncorrected poses adopted by the children when seated at the table, and in the false directions of the ideo-motor centres of which only a few reach the essential fingers that are holding or more often grotesquely clutching the pencil. It may seem a small thing to the layman that a child should try to guide a pencil by movements of its tongue, but to the expert that confusion of functions is indicative of endless subconscious troubles.

Let me describe the practical procedure of a certain type of "free-drawing" lesson. Pencils, paper, and the usual paraphernalia are placed on tables or desks in different parts of the school-room, in the hope that the child may be tempted to use them in drawing. Then, one day, a pupil takes up a pencil and makes an attempt to draw, another follows his example and so on, until all the pupils have made some kind of effort in this direction.

Now the act of drawing is in the last analysis a mechanical process that concerns the management of the fingers, and the co-ordination of the muscles of the hand and forearm in response to certain visual images conceived in the brain and imaginatively projected on to the paper. And the standard of functioning of the human fingers and hand in this connection depends entirely upon the degree of kinæsthetic development of the arm, torso, and joints; in fact upon the standard of co-ordination of the whole organism. It is not surprising, therefore, that hardly one of these more or less defectively co-ordinated children should have any idea of how to hold a pencil in such a way as will command the freedom, power, and control that will enable him to do himself justice as a draughtsman.

Any attentive and thoughtful observer who will watch the movement and position of these children's fingers, hand, wrist, arm, neck and body generally, during the varying attempts to draw straight or crooked lines, cannot fail to note the lack of co-ordination between these parts. The fingers are probably attempting to perform the duties of the arm, the shoulders are humped, the head twisted on one side. In short, energies are being projected to parts of the bodily mechanism which have little or no influence on the performance of the desired act of drawing, and the mere waste projection of such energies alone is almost sufficient to nullify the purpose in view.

But I have already said enough to prove that no free expression can come by this means. The right impulse may be in the child's mind, but he has not the physical ability to express it. Not one modern child in ten thousand is born with the gift to draw as we say "by the light of Nature," and that one exceptional child will have his task made easier if he is wisely guided in his first attempts.

So much for my two "D's," but my general criticism of the "free expression" experiment does not end there. For I must confess that I have been shocked to witness the work that has been going on in these schools.[1] I have seen children of various ages amusing themselves—somewhat inadequately in quite a number of cases—by drawing, dancing, carpentering, and so on, but in hardly a single instance have I seen an example of one of these children employing his physical mechanisms in a correct or *natural* way. I insist upon the use of the word *natural* even though it be applied to such relatively artificial activities as drawing and carpentering. For there is a right, that is to say a most effective, way of holding and using a pencil or a carpenter's tool. But the children

[1] For John Dewey's rejoinder to these comments, see Appendix I, page 171.

I saw commonly sat or stood in positions of the worst mechanical advantage, and the manner in which they held their pencils or their tools demonstrated very clearly that until their management of such instruments was corrected, they could never hope to produce anything but the most clumsy results. Worse still, these children were forming physical habits which would develop in a large majority of cases into positive physical ills. A child who tries to guide its pencil by futile movements of its head, tongue, and shoulders may be preparing the way to ills so far-reaching that their origin is often lost sight of.

Strange psychic effects may spring from apparently purely physical causes—though, indeed, the complement of psycho-physical is so unified that it is impossible to divide the components and place them on one plane or the other.

But surely I have given evidence enough to prove my case against this last development in education. In an ideal world into which children were born with ideal capacities, Mr. Shaw's thesis might have some weight. In this rapidly changing world of the 20th century we require, more than ever before, a system that shall guide and direct the child during his earlier years. This implies no contradiction of what I have said earlier anent the method of constant supervision. The necessary correction of physical and mental faults that I am advocating is a very different thing from the attempt to mould a child into one particular preconceived form. I would only insist that the children of today, born as they are with very feeble powers of instinctive control, absolutely require certain definite instructions by which to guide themselves before they can be left to free activity. And these directions must be based on a principle that will help the child to employ his various mechanisms to the best advantage in his daily activities. These directions involve no interference with what the child has to express; they represent merely a cultivation and development of the *means whereby* he may find adequate and satisfying release for his potentialities.

It is true that the foregoing principles must and will involve certain necessary prohibitions, but if we select those essentials that deal with the root cause of the evil instead of with the effects, we render unnecessary the continual admonitions and "naggings" which represented one of the vices of the old system, a vice from which it has been the object of the new education to free the child.

To sum up this aspect of child-training, I find that on the whole the methods of the older educationalists, with their definite prohibitions and their exact instructions, were less harmful than the extremes of the modern school that would base their scheme of education upon a child's instinctive reactions. The older methods failed, I admit, for one reason, because the system was carried too far; for another, because the injunctions and prohibitions were based on tradition, prejudice, and ignorance, instead of upon a scientific principle dictated by reason. But the new methods fail because they are founded on an entirely erroneous assumption which is demonstrably fallacious. Can any method be defended that is open to such a charge?

Give a child conscious control and you give him poise, the essential starting point for education. Without that poise, which is a result aimed at by neither the old nor the new methods of education, he will presently be cramped and distorted by his environment. For although you may choose the environment of a nursery or a school, there are few, indeed, who can choose their desired environment in the world at large. But give the child poise and the reasoned control of his physical being and you fit him for any and every mode of life; he will have wonderful powers of adapting himself to any and every environment that may surround him. And if he be one of those exceptional individuals that, by some rare gift of nature or by some force of personality, are able to bend life to their own needs, be very sure that so far from having suppressed his power of free expression, you will have strengthened and perfected just those abilities which will enable the genius to put forth all that is best and greatest in him.

My last charge against the advocates of free expression is that they themselves are not free. So many propagandists and teachers show an unwarranted intolerance towards the exponents of the old systems. They are, in fact, too constricted in their mental attitude to give play to their imagination. From one extreme they have flown to the other, and so have missed the way of the great middle course which is wide enough to accommodate all shades of opinion.

For let me state clearly in concluding this comment on a new method, that I am, myself, as strong an advocate for free expression, rightly understood, as any propagandist in the United States of America. But I am convinced by long observation and experiment that the untrained child has not the adequate power of free expression. There are certain mechanical and other laws, deduced from untold centuries of human experience, laws that are only in the rarest cases unconsciously followed by the natural child of today.

Over twenty-two years ago in Australia, I was teaching what I still believe to be the true meaning of free expression. My pupils in this case came to me for lessons in vocal and dramatic expression. Now by the old methods these pupils would have been taught to imitate their master very accurately in vocal and facial expression, in gesture, in the manner of voice production; and it would have been at once apparent to any one acquainted with the manner and methods of the teachers, where each pupil had received his training. Furthermore, pupils educated by those methods were taught to interpret each poem, scene, or passage on the exact lines that were considered correct by their respective teachers.

My own method, which at that time was regarded as very radical and subversive, was to give my pupils certain lessons in re-education and co-ordination on a basis of conscious guidance and control, and in this way I gave the reciter, actor, or potential artist the means of employing to the best advantage his powers of vocal, facial, and dramatic expression, gesture, etc. He could then safely be permitted to develop his own characteristics. A few suggestions might be necessary as to interpretation, but the individual manner was his own. No pupil of mine could be pointed to as representing some narrow school of expression, although most of them could be recognized by the confidence and freedom of their performances.

And in this connection it may be of interest to my readers to know that in 1902–3 I decided to test the principles I advocated, and to this end I organized performances of "Hamlet" and "The Merchant of Venice" for which I gave special training on the lines I have just indicated to young men and women, none of whom had previously appeared in a public performance of any kind whatsoever. I trained all these young people on the principles of conscious guidance and control, principles that I had then developed and practised. My friends and critics naturally anticipated a wonderful exhibition of "stage fright" on the evening of the first performance, but as a matter of fact not one of my young students had the least apprehension of that terror. By the time they were ready to appear the idea of "stage fright" was one that seemed to them the merest absurdity. It may be said that they did not understand what was meant by such a condition. And this, although I would not allow a prompter on the nights of the public performances! I regard this as one of the most convincing public demonstrations I have yet made of the wonderful command and self-possession that may be attained by the inculcation of these principles.

For it must be observed that I sent these tyros to the performance capable of expressing their own individualities. If they had been hedged about or boxed in by an endless series of "Don'ts" confining their performances by a rigid set of rules, the majority of them would almost certainly have broken down within the first two minutes. On the other hand, it is hardly necessary to picture the chaos that would have ensued, had I sent them on the stage without training of any kind, poor, helpless, ignorant examples of what they supposed to be free expression.

The foregoing is an example of education in only one sphere of art, but it serves as an excellent indication of the essential needs of education, in general, where the child is concerned. We must give the child of today and of the future as a fundamental of education as complete a command of his or her kinæsthetic systems as is possible, so that the highest possible standard of "free expression" may be given in every sphere of life and in all forms of human activity. We must build up, co-ordinate, and readjust the human machine so that it may be *in tune*.

It is said that the dividing line between tragedy and comedy is not one that the majority of people readily recognize, and this is also the case in regard to what is called freedom and licence. This is the danger which the new democracies of the world are facing at this very moment, and their dangers will be increased a thousandfold in the near future, when they will be called upon to pass through that critical period of re-adjustment which must follow the present world crisis.

In this matter of education I am, admittedly an iconoclast. I would fain break down the idols of tradition and set up new concepts. In no matter do we see more plainly the harmful effect of the rigid convention than in this matter of teaching. We speak commonly of training the minds of children. It is a happy expression in its origin, and we still retain its proper intention when we apply the word to its uses in horticulture.

The gardener does, indeed, train the young growth. He draws it out to the light and warmth and leads it into the conditions most helpful for its development.

And so, in teaching, the first essential should be to cultivate the uses of the mind and body, and not, as is so often the case, to neglect the instrument of thought and reason by the inculcation of fixed rules which have never been examined. Again, where ideas that are patently erroneous have already been formed in the child's mind, the teacher should take pains to apprehend these preconceptions, and in dealing with them he should not attempt to overlay them, but should eradicate them as far as possible before teaching or submitting the new and correct idea. I say "teaching or submitting" and perhaps the latter word better expresses my meaning, for by teaching I understand the placing of facts, for and against, before the child, in such a way as to appeal to his reasoning faculties, and to his latent powers of originality. He should be allowed to think for himself, and should not be crammed with other people's ideas, or one side only of a controversial subject. Why should not the child's powers of intelligence be trained? Why should they be stunted by our forcing him to accept the preconceived ideas and traditions which have been handed down from generation to generation, without examination, without reason, *without enquiry as to their truth or origin?* The human mind of today is suffering from partial paralysis by this method of forcing these unreasoned and antiquated principles upon the young and plastic intelligence.

*Chapter Three*

# THE TROUBLE WITH
# PHYSICAL EXERCISES

In Australia over forty years ago, in the rooms of one of the best teachers of physical culture I have ever known, I had my first experience of observing the results of exercises designed to bring about "specific effects." Although I disagreed then, as I still do, with the principle underlying his and all such teaching, we were both impressed by the fact that *the same set of exercises was responsible for quite different effects in different people.* How could it be otherwise?

We all notice differences in people's manner of walking and speaking, and this same difference in use they bring to the performance of the exercises. The specific effect desired, as well as the by-products of one exercise or more, will not be exactly the same in any two people, and if this be so, who is to decide which of the exercises—whether all or only a selected few—are to be used, and in what order they are to be practised if they are to meet the variations in kind of the various mal-conditions which in most people create the need for the "desired physical development"?

For years past I have drawn the attention of medical men to the evils wrought by the physical training and the "stand-at-attention" attitude in vogue in the army, and also to the harmful effects of the drill in our schools, where the unfortunate children are made to assume a posture which is exactly that of the soldier, whose striking characteristic is the undue and harmful hollow in the lumbar spine and the numerous defects that are inseparable from this unnatural posture.

How consistently both by precept and example, wrong values in matters of physical culture are now being inculcated upon the general public! Surely a university boat race should be a friendly contest between men animated by the sporting instinct. Every one of them should wish the victory to go to the best crew. It should be an experience of pleasure, happiness and healthy recreation to

109

all concerned, not an unnatural struggle involving distortion and loss of consciousness through the "determination" to gain an end even at the cost of personal exhaustion and damage. What difference does it really make in the long run whether or not an Oxford or Cambridge crew wins the boat race in a particular year? None whatever—people indulging in sport today whether it be rowing, football, cricket or what-not, seem to be losing all sense of proportion, all idea of relative values. In the interest of all concerned, it were far better if we engaged in sport for sport's sake.

Now what I wish to emphasize is that throughout the long search for the remedy for his deterioration, man overlooked certain most important factors in the case, factors which are still overlooked today by the majority of people in their search for health and general uplifting.

In the first place, man completely overlooked the fact that the sensory mechanism, upon which he had heretofore entirely depended for guidance in general activity, was no longer registering accurately, and that he could no longer rely, therefore, entirely upon feeling, that is, on instinctive subconscious guidance for the satisfactory performance of the ordinary acts of life. The very fact that at some period "physical exercises" were considered necessary proves that imperfections must have developed to a very serious extent, and the reason for this, as I again repeat, is that the gradual failure of the sense registers to continue to guide men satisfactorily in the use of themselves in the activities of life had finally brought about an advanced stage of mal-co-ordination in the human psycho-physical organism.

It was clearly unreasonable, therefore, to expect "physical exercises" of whatever kind, to bring about any lasting or fundamental improvement in this unsatisfactory condition, when the person performing them would be guided by the same imperfect and delusive sensory appreciation, *dependence upon which had led originally to the very condition he wished to remedy.* What is more, during the performance of "physical exercises" under these conditions there would be an actual development of his original mal-co-ordinated condition, and he would be sure to encounter some new and very baffling psycho-physical problems in himself. These problems actually arose and have become since then increasingly complicated, and I should like here to reiterate that even if they cannot be said to be wholly overlooked today, their real significance is still almost entirely misunderstood, in that the majority of people do not realize that human beings are still propelling an already maladjusted and damaged mechanism along the difficult road of modern life, whilst relying for guidance upon an imperfect and sometimes delusive sensory appreciation.

Secondly, in choosing "physical exercises" as a remedy for his deterioration, man did not take into consideration the fact that his body was a very delicate and highly co-ordinated piece of machinery, so that there might be many contributing causes other than muscular weakness to account for his deteriorated condition; further, that the exercises themselves were not correlated in any way to the needs of his organism, either in the practical activities of life or during those periods of rest which are such an important part of the daily round (a point constantly overlooked by enthusiasts for "physical culture").

If we ask ourselves why man overlooked these important points, the answer may throw light on many of our own problems at the present time. It was undoubtedly because he was aiming exclusively at a method of "cure," not of prevention. In the terms of my thesis, his attention was fixed on the "end" he was seeking (his "physical" amelioration), not on the reasonable *means whereby* that "end" could be brought about.

If he could have thought of his body in the terms of the very intricately constructed machine which it is, he would have seen in his deteriorated condition, not a deterioration in his muscular development alone, but a deterioration in his general psycho-physical co-ordination, accompanied by an interference with the general adjustment of the organism and by a general lowering of the standard of its functioning. He would then have realized that his deterioration must be merely the symptom of some failure in the working of the machinery, *and that the whole machine would need to be readjusted before it could work co-ordinately once more.*

He would have dealt with it as he would have dealt with any other machine, his watch, for instance, that was out of working order. If his watch gained half an hour one day and on the next stopped altogether, or if its small hand worked at the same speed as the big one, he would not trust to its accuracy if he wanted to catch a train, and, still more to the point, he would not start to repair it at random. He would send it instead to an expert who, through his knowledge of the correct working of the machinery, would make good any worn or broken part and readjust the mechanism once more. The watchmaker would then probably suggest, *as a preventive measure,* a periodic overhaul so that wear might be watched, and, when necessary, damaged parts repaired or new ones supplied. By this means, a reasonable endeavour would be made to *prevent* another such derangement of the mechanism as had rendered the watch an unreliable guide.[1]

We cannot be surprised, however, that man did not reason in the same way in connexion with the deterioration of his own mechanism. His reasoning processes in connexion with the care of his own mechanisms and with his general well-being had not been employed to anything like the same degree as in connexion with the mechanisms of external nature. He decided that he had discovered a "physical" defect for which he must find a remedy, and there can be little doubt that as soon as he conceived the "remedy" idea, any other possible consideration was shut off, whether of the cause or causes of the "physical" deterioration, or of the psychophysical principles involved, or (even if the cause or causes had been discovered), of the *means whereby* the desired "end" (remedy) could be secured. His decision, in short, was the result of a subconscious and, therefore, unreasoned procedure, not of conscious reasoning reflexion. As we have already pointed out, a different result could hardly be expected at this early stage of man's development, seeing that even to-day in the twentieth century, the problem of psycho-physical unfitness is met with the same primeval "remedy" outlook both in theory and practice.

The stubborn but unpleasant fact must be faced that civilized man has never progressed personally, that is, in himself, as he has

[1] We must again note the difference that exists between human and inanimate machinery. The human machine, when in a state of co-ordinated and adequate use, commands in itself the power of growth and development in each part of the muscular mechanism, and the condition approximating to wear in inanimate machinery may be prevented more or less from becoming present in the human being by nature's method of supply and repair under right conditions in the matter of used and wasted tissue.

advanced in matters outside himself. Although he has reasoned out the *means whereby* he can control and turn to his own uses the different forces he has discovered in the outside world, he has not applied this reasoning principle where his own organism is concerned. He has left this masterpiece of psycho-physical machinery, more subtle, more delicate in its workings than the most intricate man-made machine, to the subconscious guidance of his sensory appreciation, unaware that this sensory appreciation is becoming, as we have seen, more and more unreliable with the boasted advance of civilization.

## Chapter Four

# ABOUT GOLF

Let us suppose that a golfer who does not make a success of his golf consults a professional with a view to improving his play. After watching him play, the professional tells him among other things that he is taking his eyes off the ball, and impresses on him that if he wishes to improve his stroke, he *must* keep his eyes on the ball. The golfer starts to play with every intention of following out his teacher's instructions, but finds that in spite of all his efforts, he still takes his eyes off the ball.

There are several points in this situation that could be discussed, but I wish, in this chapter, to confine my consideration to the principle which underlies not only the teacher's diagnosis and instructions, but also the procedure of the pupil when he decides to carry the instructions out.

Certain questions at once suggest themselves.

Why does the golfer take his eyes off the ball in the first place, when according to the experts he should not do so?

Why does he *continue* to take his eyes off the ball after he has decided to keep them *on* the ball? Why does his "will to do" fail him at the critical moment?

What is the stimulus that constitutes an apparently irresistible temptation to him to take his eyes off the ball, in spite of his desire to follow his teacher's instructions and in spite of his "will to do"?

To answer these questions we shall have to take them in their connexion with each other, for the answers are as closely related to one another as the questions are themselves.

To take the first question.

When the golfer starts to make his stroke, he brings to the act the same habitual use of his mechanisms that he brings to all his activities, and since for such an essential part of the recognized golfing technique as "keeping his eyes on the ball" the mechanisms concerned with the control of his eyes fail to function as he desires, we are justified in concluding that his habitual use is misdirected. This fact is practically admitted by the instructor when he attributes

115

his pupil's failure to make a good stroke to his failure to keep his eyes on the ball.[1]

To the question why he continues to take his eyes off the ball, in spite of his intention to follow his teacher's instructions and in spite of his "will to do," the answer is that in everything he does he is a confirmed "end-gainer." His habit is to work directly for his ends on the "trial and error" plan without giving due consideration to the means whereby those ends should be gained. In the present instance there can be no doubt that the particular end he has in view is to make a good stroke, which means that the moment he begins to play he starts to work for that end directly, without considering what manner of use of his mechanisms generally would be the best for the making of a good stroke. The result is that he makes the stroke according to his habitual use, and as this habitual use is misdirected and includes the wrong use of his eyes, he takes his eyes off the ball and makes a bad stroke. It is clear that as long as he is dominated by his habit of end-gaining, he will react to the stimulus to "make a good stroke" by the same misdirected use of himself, and will continue to take his eyes off the ball.

This process is repeated every time he tries to make a good stroke, with the result that his failures far outnumber his successes, and he becomes more or less disturbed emotionally,[2] as always happens when people find themselves more often wrong than not, without knowing the reason why. And the more he finds himself unable to carry out his teacher's instructions with anything like the necessary degree of certainty for him to get any pleasure out of the game, the worse this emotional condition becomes. The immediate effect is that he tries harder than ever to make a good stroke, falls into the old wrong way of using his mechanisms, and again takes his eyes off the ball.

Now one would suppose that repeated experience of failure

[1] I admit, of course, that a wrong use of other parts might have a more direct bearing upon the golfer's problem, but for the purpose of illustration I have chosen the wrong use of the eyes, because the experts are unanimously agreed (as unanimously as experts ever are) that failure to keep the eyes on the ball is one of the most common and persistent hindrances to the making of a good stroke.

[2] Unsuccessful effort in any sphere of activity tends to produce emotional disturbance which is not conducive to healthy recreation. For this reason alone the golfer whose efforts to carry out his teacher's instructions are mostly unsuccessful should reconsider his plan of campaign.

would of itself lead him to set to work on a different principle, but my teaching experience goes to shew that in this respect the golfer's method of procedure is in no way different from that of other people who use themselves wrongly, and who are trying, without success, to correct a defect. Strange as it may seem, I have always found that a pupil who uses himself wrongly will continue to do so in all his activities, even after the wrong use has been pointed out to him, and he has learned by experience that persistence in this wrong use is the cause of his failure.

This apparent anomaly can be explained, and in explaining it I hope to shew not only what is at the bottom of the golfer's difficulty, but also of the difficulty which so many people experience when, with the best "will" in the world, they find themselves unable to put right something which they know to be wrong with themselves.

The habitual use of his mechanisms which the golfer brings to all his activities, including golf, has always been accompanied by certain sensory experiences (feelings) which, from their lifelong association with this habitual use, have become familiar to him. Further, from their very familiarity, they have come to "feel right," and so he derives considerable satisfaction from repeating them. When, therefore, he attempts to "make a good stroke," he brings to the act of swinging his club his faulty habitual use, including the taking of his eyes off the ball, because the sensory experiences associated with this use are familiar and "feel right."

On the other hand, the use of his mechanisms which would involve his keeping his eyes *on* the ball during the act of making a stroke would be a use entirely contrary to his habitual use and associated with *sensory experiences which, being unfamiliar, would "feel wrong" to him;* it may therefore be said that he receives no sensory stimulus in that direction. Any sensory stimulus he receives is in the direction of repeating the familiar sensory experiences which accompany his faulty use, and this carries the day over any so-called "mental" stimulus arising from his "will to do." In other words, the lure of the familiar proves too strong for him and keeps him tied down to the habitual use of himself which *feels right.*

This is not surprising, seeing that the golfer's desire to employ his habitual use at all costs in gaining his end, on account of the familiar sensory experiences that go with it, is an instinctive desire which mankind has inherited and continued to develop all through the ages. *The desire to feel right in the gaining of his end* is therefore his primary desire, in comparison with which his desire to make a good stroke is new and undeveloped, and exerts only a secondary influence. This is proved by the fact that although he starts out with the desire to make a good stroke, his desire to repeat sensory experiences that "feel right" acts as a stimulus to him to use himself in the habitual way which is associated with these experiences, although it is this very manner of use that prevents him from satisfying his newer desire to make a good stroke.

The desire to carry out his teacher's instructions to keep his eyes on the ball is a still newer desire, and consequently suffers in intensity as compared with the other two. Moreover, it stands even less chance of being carried out, firstly, because the stimulus which gives rise to it does not come from within, like the others, but from without, i.e., from the teacher, and secondly, because the instruction is framed with the purpose of correcting something wrong with the pupil's use, i.e., the use of the eyes, and so is bound to come at once into conflict with the pupil's desire to employ his faulty habitual use which, as we have just explained, is the dominating influence in whatever he tries to do. The conflict between these two desires is therefore bound to be an unequal one, and his desire to carry out his teacher's instructions goes by the board.[1]

It is the dominating influence of his desire to gain his end by means of a use of his mechanisms which *feels* right, but is in fact wrong for the purpose, that explains not only why he *continues* to take his eyes off the ball and so to fail in his stroke, but also why, in spite of this repeated experience of failure, he does not give up "end-gaining" and set to work in a different way.

Now that we have seen the faulty principle which underlies the golfer's efforts to obey his teacher's instructions, we will go on to examine the principle on which these instructions are based.

The instruction to the pupil to "keep his eyes on the ball"

[1] It must be remembered that the greater his desire to obey his teacher, the greater will be his incentive to increase the intensity of his efforts, and it is practically certain that in his attempts to translate this desire into action, he will automatically increase the already undue muscle tension which he habitually employs for the act, thus lessening still further his chances of making a successful stroke.

shews that the teacher recognizes that the mechanisms concerned with the control of the pupil's eyes do not function as they should, but when, in order to meet this difficulty, he simply tells his pupil to "keep his eyes on the ball," he also shews that he does not connect the faulty functioning of the eyes with misdirection of the use of the mechanisms throughout the organism. This means that in his diagnosis and treatment he is not considering his pupil's organism as a working unity in which the working of any of the parts is affected by the working of the whole. To this extent, therefore, the diagnosis may be said to be incomplete and his scope of usefulness as adviser to his pupil limited.

Evidence of misdirection of use in human activity is to be found on all sides, and our real interest in the golfer's difficulty is that it is a difficulty not confined to golf, but experienced by all who are trying, without success, to correct defects which hamper them in their various activities, or to perform a certain act satisfactorily.

Misdirection of use is to be found in the person who takes up a pen to write and proceeds at once to stiffen the fingers unduly, to make movements of the arm which should be made by the fingers, and even to make facial contortions; in the physical culturist whose performance of certain movements of the arms or legs, or of both, is associated with harmful and unnecessary depression of the larynx and with undue tension of the musculature of the thorax; in the person who in reading or singing or talking "sucks" a breath in through the mouth at the beginning of each sentence, though in the ordinary way, in walking or standing, he would breathe through the nostrils; in the athlete, amateur or professional, who, whenever he makes a special effort, employs excessive tension in the muscles of the neck and pulls the head back unduly.

In all these cases, which might be elaborated indefinitely, it will be found that the use of the mechanisms concerned with the movement required is often far removed from that which would best serve the purpose.

This all goes to shew that in every form of activity the use of the mechanisms which come into operation will be satisfactory or unsatisfactory according to whether our direction of that use is satisfactory or otherwise. Where the direction is satisfactory, satisfactory use of the mechanisms of the organism as a working unity will be ensured, involving a satisfactory use of the different parts, such as the arms, wrists, hands, legs, feet and eyes. It follows that where there is misdirection, this satisfactory use of the mechanisms is not at our command. This is exactly the position of the golfer who cannot keep his eyes on the ball when he desires.

Let us now see how the golfer's difficulty would be dealt with by a teacher who adhered to the idea of the unity of the organism, and so based his teaching practice on what I call the "means-whereby" principle, i.e., the principle of a reasoning consideration of the causes of the conditions present, and an indirect instead of a direct procedure on the part of the person endeavouring to gain the desired end.

First he would diagnose the golfer's failure to make a good stroke as due to misdirection of the habitual use of the mechanisms, and not primarily to any specific defect such as an inability to keep the eyes on the ball. He would recognize that the inability to keep the eyes on the ball was merely a symptom of this misdirection, and could not by any stretch of imagination be said to be the cause of his failure to make a good stroke. He would observe that im-mediately his pupil started to make his stroke, he brought into play the same faulty use which he habitually employed for all his activities, and so himself brought about the very thing he wanted to prevent, the taking of his eyes off the ball. He would see that his pupil's difficulty was to a great extent caused by his own "wrong-doing."

A teacher who made a diagnosis on these lines would under-stand that the difficulty could not be met by any such purely specific instruction as telling his pupil to keep his eyes on the ball, for he would recognize that any "will power" exerted by a pupil whose use of himself was misdirected would be exerted in the wrong direction,[1] so that the harder he tried to carry out such an instruc-

---

[1] Not long ago a professor brought a friend to watch a lesson given to one of his students in whose progress they were both interested on account of her attain-ments. "You should have no difficulty with this pupil," he said, "because she is so willing and anxious to help you." "Yes," I replied, "that is one of the curses of the 'will to do.'" His companion held up her hands in horror at this, exclaiming, "Surely, even if it's wrong, it's better to exert the 'will to do' than not." This gave me the chance to point out that the "something wrong" meant that there was a wrong direction somewhere, so that what she was really urging was that the addition of the stimulus of the "will to do" would be beneficial, even though it

tion and the more he "willed" himself to succeed, the more his use would be misdirected and the more likely he would be to take his eyes off the ball. From this he would conclude that he must find some way of teaching his pupil to stop the misdirection of his use, and as he observed that the misdirection began the moment the pupil tried to gain his end and make a good stroke, obviously his first step would be to get the pupil to stop "trying to make a good stroke." He would explain that any immediate reaction to the stimulus to make a good stroke would always be by means of his wrong habitual use, but that if he prevented this immediate reaction, he would at the same time be preventing the misdirection of his use that went with it and was *the* obstacle to the gaining of his end. He would impress upon him that of all the activities that go to the making of a good stroke, *this act of prevention was the primary activity,* since by the inhibition of the misdirected habitual use the way would be left clear for the teacher to build up in his pupil that new direction of the use of his mechanisms, which would constitute the means whereby he would in time be able to keep his eyes on the ball, and thus make a good stroke.

---

involved an increased projection of energy in the wrong direction. It is not the degree of "willing" or "trying," *but the way* in which the energy is directed, that is going to make the "willing" or "trying" effective.

# FEAR, PREJUDICE AND
# OTHER EMOTIONAL STATES

There can be little doubt that the process of reasoning tends to develop more quickly and to reach a higher standard in a person whose attitude towards life might be described as calm and collected. In such a person, the psycho-physical processes called "habits" are governed by moderation, and his inhibitory processes are adequately developed in all spheres of activity. Their use is not limited to those comparatively few spheres where it was considered necessary to establish taboos during the early and later periods of man's struggle with the problems which arose in the various stages of the civilizing process. In these spheres there has been a harmful and exaggerated development of the inhibitory processes, often causing virtues to become almost vices, whilst in other spheres there has been a correspondingly harmful lack of the development of inhibition, particularly in those spheres connected with the use of the psycho-physical mechanisms in practical activity. This represents an unbalanced use of this wonderful process of inhibition, and tends to produce, as a general result, a state of unbalanced psycho-physical functioning throughout the whole organism, and to establish what we shall refer to as "the unduly excited reflex" process.

This unbalanced psycho-physical condition of the civilized human creature is apparent in most spheres of activity, and the child of to-day is more predisposed to the factors which make for this condition than his parents or their ancestors. This child, therefore, starts his school career with a comparatively poor equipment on the inhibitory side. Now volition and inhibition are invaluable birthrights of the human creature and should be developed equally, as it were, hand in hand, but from the first moment of a child's school life right on to adolescence the training[1] he receives tends

[1] The fact of the great number of "don'ts" to which some children are subjected, and the implicit obedience expected of them at school and at home, does not affect my contention that the children of to-day manifest a serious lack on the inhibitory side in all activity involving the use of the psycho-physical organism.

to interfere with his balanced development, and so is another factor in the cultivation of those psycho-physical defects and abnormalities which make for the unbalanced condition to which we have already referred.

Unduly excited fear reflexes, uncontrolled emotions, prejudices and fixed habits, are retarding factors in all human development. They need our serious attention, for they are linked up with all psycho-physical processes employed in growth and development on the subconscious plane. Hence, by the time adolescence is reached, these retarding factors have become present in a more or less degree, and the processes thus established in psycho-physical use will make for the continued development of such retarding factors. This is particularly the case when a person endeavours to learn something calling for new experiences.

It is only necessary to watch adult pupils at their lessons to realize that, in the great majority of cases, more or less uncontrolled emotions are a striking feature in their endeavours to carry out new instructions correctly. Watch the fixed expression of these pupils, for instance, their jerky, uncontrolled movements, and their tendency to hold the breath by assuming a harmful posture and exerting an exaggerated strain such as they would employ in performing strenuous "physical" acts. In many cases there will be a twitching of the muscles of the mouth and cheeks, or of the fingers. In each case, the stimulus to these misdirected activities is the pupil's idea or conception that he must try to do *correctly* whatever the teacher requests, and, as we have seen, on the subconscious plane the teacher insists upon this. The teacher of re-education on a conscious plane does not make this demand of his pupils, for he knows by experience, and has to face the fact that in cases where there is an imperfect functioning of the organism, *an individual cannot always do as he is told correctly*. He may "want" to do it, he may "try and try again" to do it, but as long as the psycho-mechanics by which he tries to carry out his teacher's directions are not working satisfactorily, every attempt he makes to carry out his teacher's directions "correctly" (trying to be right) is bound to end in comparative failure. For in making these attempts, as we point out elsewhere, the pupil has only his own judgment to depend on as to what is correct, and since his judgment is based on incorrect direction and delusive sensory appreciation, he is held within the vicious circle of his old habits as long as he tries to carry out the directions "correctly." Paradoxical as it may seem, the pupil's only chance of success lies, not in "trying to be right," but, on the contrary, in "wanting to be wrong," wrong, that is, according to any standard of his own. In this connexion, it is most important to remember that every unsuccessful "try" not only reinforces the pupil's old wrong psycho-physical habits associated with his conception of a particular act, but involves at the same time new emotional experiences of discouragement, worry, fear, and anxiety, so that the wrong experiences and the unduly excited reflex process involved in these experiences become one in the pupil's recognition; they "make the meat they feed on," and the more conscientious the teacher and the pupil are on this plane, the worse the situation becomes for both.

It is for this reason that the teacher on a conscious plane does not expect a pupil, as I have pointed out, to perform "correctly" a new act calling for new experiences, but instead, by means of manipulation, gives to the pupil the new experiences, repeating them until they become established. Indeed, a process which does not involve a pupil's being asked to perform any act, until his teacher has prepared the way by raising the standard of the pupil's sensory appreciation and psycho-physical co-ordination to that satisfactory state which will enable him to perform the act, as we say, easily, will be a process which ensures that the pupil's experiences will be, with rare exceptions, satisfactory experiences, which make for confidence and are not associated with those emotional disturbances which tend towards the minimum instead of the maximum functioning.

The relation of all this to the very important question of the ability to "keep one's head" at critical moments is clear, and it may be interesting to apply the points we have raised in the foregoing to such activities as playing games and to other performances in which skill and so-called "presence of mind" are required. We constantly hear in this connexion remarks like the following: "I didn't do so badly at it at first, but the longer I play the worse I play." One writer in the public Press remarks that it is a curious feature of golf that "the more one knows about it . . . the more difficult it seems to become"; and another writes that a well-known professional had "confessed . . . that golf had become almost too much for him." All this applies equally, of course, to other games, but I have chosen golf for my illustration because it happens that writers on golf, commenting on some of the incidents that have occurred at matches during the past two years or so, have unwittingly emphasized the existence of *the problem* which underlies these admissions and with which I am dealing in the present book. For instance, they have commented on the failure of certain experts to perform some simple stroke when under an unusual stress, and at a moment when success depends on their not throwing a chance away; they have pointed to the tendency of some players to become confused and to hurry their strokes through anxiety to "get it over"; "truly heart-breaking" is the description of one such incident, words that will be echoed by many who have had similar discouraging experiences in other matters besides golf.

We are told that this is all a matter of "nerves" and so forth. It is undoubtedly a case of the undue excitement of fear reflexes on the player's part, fear, for instance, that he may miss a shot which he knows he is not in the habit of missing and ought not to miss. As a pupil once said to me at a first interview, "I am always coming up against things that I know I can do, and yet when it comes to the point, I can't do them." The fact is that in all our processes of learning things, the fear reflexes are unduly and harmfully excited by the teaching methods employed, according to which demands are made upon us that we are not able to fulfil. So, for a time, we get bad results, with the undue and harmful development of emotional reflex processes which, as we have seen, inevitably accompanies these unsuccessful attempts. We continue to practise on wrong lines, so that our successful experiences are few and our unsuccessful experiences many. We attempt on a subconscious basis to develop a particular stroke, and in any failure to make the stroke satisfactorily the imperfect use of the psycho-physical mechanisms plays more than its fair share. It is experiences like this which cause disappointment and undue excitement of fear reflexes and serious emotional disturbances, and nothing whatever is done at this later stage of the process to nullify these effects of the psycho-physical experiences cultivated during the earlier stages.

These emotional disturbances were part and parcel of an unbalanced psycho-physical condition, of a state of anxiety and confusion, and there can be little doubt that any circumstance that is more or less unusual is likely to bring about a recurrence of the same disturbed psycho-physical condition as was experienced by the subject during his early efforts to make the stroke.

But, beyond this, we must remember that it is only the small minority of experts in any line who really know *how* they get their results and effects, in the case of golf, for instance, *how* they perform their most successful strokes. Therefore directly anything puts them "off their game," they experience considerable difficulty, at any rate, in getting on to it again. It is only by having a clear conception of what is required for the successful performance of a certain stroke or other act, combined with a knowledge of the psycho-physical *means whereby* those requirements can be met, that there is any reasonable possibility of their attaining sureness and confidence during performance.

We must realize that if an individual is to reach that satisfactory stage of progress where he can be reasonably certain of success in achieving his "ends," those principles must be observed which imply reliance in all activities upon the *means whereby* an "end" may be gained, irrespective of whether, during the progress of the activities concerned, the performance is correct or incorrect. The application of these principles in any sphere of learning means that the teacher during lessons must be able to supply the pupil's needs in the matter of reliable sensory appreciation, by giving him from day to day the necessary experiences until they become established. No technique which does not meet the demands herein indicated will prove satisfactory as a means of re-educating a pupil on a general basis to a reliable plane of conscious activity. When this plane is reached, the individual comes to rely upon his "means-whereby," and does not become disturbed by wondering whether the activities concerned will be right or wrong. Why should he, seeing that the confidence with which he proceeds with his task is a confidence born of experiences, the majority of which are successful experiences unassociated with over-excited fear reflexes? This confidence is further reinforced by his confidence in the reliability of his sensory appreciation which ensures that any interference with the co-ordinated use of himself will come to his consciousness as soon as it occurs (awareness). This consciousness is really a state of acute awareness which has been developed in him during the processes of re-education and co-ordination on a general basis, and the confidence associated with it is not likely to desert him in moments of crisis. It is true that he may be put off the right track, but he knows that it will only be momentarily, as he is certain that his awareness, associated as it is with reliable sensory appreciation, will not fail him in such situations or crises, but will prove his protector and reliable guide; for this state of awareness means that he will be able at such moments to remember, reason and judge (that is, to size up the situation, as we say), and the resultant judgment, based as it is upon experiences associated with reliable sensory appreciation and unassociated with unduly excited fear reflexes, will be in its turn a sound and reliable judgment.

This matter of unduly excited fear reflexes has been referred to in connexion with education and here I wish to discuss processes used in tests made on children.

In some schools special mechanical tests are made in order to discover the potentialities and qualities of the children and to grade them accordingly. The young and undeveloped organism of the child's "mental apparatus" is, as it were, put upon the rack, and his intellectual status and probably his educational fate depend upon the result of these tests which are supposed to be a reliable guide, not only as to the line of procedure to be taken in regard to the details of his school education, but also as to the particular career for which he will be best adapted when the state of adolescence is reached.

A teacher recently told me of an interesting personal experience in this connexion. She visited a modern school where a psychologist was engaged in testing the children for such qualities as accuracy, muscular control, observation, etc. She was taken into a small room set apart for the purpose of such tests. A boy of seven was waiting there to be tested for "control." He had shewn various symptoms which were described as "nervous," and the test to be taken was to enable the school authorities to prescribe a curriculum to meet his special needs. The test was made as follows. An apparatus, electrically worked, was placed in front of the child. It consisted of a metal tray in which were sunk two rows of shallow circular holes decreasing gradually in size from that of a shilling to a very small size. The boy was told to touch the centre of each hole with a small metal rod tapering to a point like a pencil. If he made a mistake and touched the side of a hole in his effort to get the centre, an electric flash would be the result.

The child, so I was told, was already in a state of nervous dread, and when he received the instruction, "Now you must try and touch the centre of each hole, and do not touch the side of any hole or else you will make a flash," he at once became so excited *through the fear of making a mistake* that his hand shook and he stiffened and tensed his whole body unduly in making the first try. He was therefore unable to control his hand to find the centre of the first hole, touched the side and produced a flash. Still more frightened by this, still more anxious not to do the wrong thing again, he proceeded from hole to hole, making flash after flash, realizing that every mistake he made was being noted by the "tester," against him, as he thought, so that, by the time he had reached the last hole his condition was one of undue excitement. It is obvious that a test taken with such emotional conditions present was not a reliable test of his control or a trustworthy guide to anyone wishing to estimate his potentialities and general qualities. Indeed, I am prepared to prove by demonstration that nine out of ten of the children now being submitted to tests are imperfectly co-ordinated, and that a great number are beset with very serious psycho-physical defects.

Where the imperfectly co-ordinated child is concerned, its first need is to be readjusted and coordinated on a plane of conscious control, until the standard of functioning in psycho-physical use of the organism is adequate. The organism will then function as near to the maximum as is possible, and the potentialities for improved functioning will continue as the child gradually develops to that standard of conscious guidance and control in psycho-physical use, which makes for the conditions essential to the fullest development of latent potentialities.

.        .        .        .        .

We have all heard instances advanced of wonderful feats being performed by people in an emotional state, of "faith cures" being effected when the subjects of these "cures" are in that uncontrolled and harmful psycho-physical state which is akin to conditions associated with drunkenness, and which at times approximates to mild insanity. For instance, the writer was acquainted with a man who never accomplished anything worth mentioning in his particular sphere of life until he was half crazed with alcohol. He also knows of a carriage painter who is unable to put in the straight lines satisfactorily unless he is well under the influence of alcohol. We can all point to instances of men and women who have performed remarkable acts whilst in an uncontrolled emotional state, in which they have been a danger to themselves and to those around them. Men are sent into battle in a half-drunken condition in order that their "controls" may be temporarily released, and for centuries bands of musicians have been employed in warfare to induce this emotional condition of lowered control. "Muddling through by instinct" is unintelligent enough, but deliberately to induce in human beings by artificial means, (such as the processes involved in methods of "faith cure," auto-suggestion, religious revivalism, etc.), a condition of lowered control, where intelligence and reasoning are superseded by uncontrolled emotions, is a procedure which may be described as an insult to even a very lowly evolved intelligence. All concerned reach the borderland of insanity through the use of such means for the accomplishment of their aims, and the psycho-physical experiences involved have only to be repeated sufficiently to bring madness in their train. In all these instances, the "end-gaining" principle is in operation, and the people subjected to these unnatural and harmful experiences are more or less influenced by them in after life, for the uncontrolled forces which run riot on these occasions are rarely mastered again, and recur more or less in other spheres of activity, frequently developing into dangerous manifestations, culminating often in tragedy. Small wonder that after the experience of 1914–1918 we are confronted with dangerous uncontrolled forces in human activity which, before the War, were manifested only by a small minority! When the individual is dominated by his uncontrolled emotions, even a weak stimulus will often cause him to indulge in dangerous activities, leading him temporarily to experiences which are well within the psycho-physical state which we call "insanity." The repetition of such experiences is the beginning of the formation of what we call a habit, in this case, the habit of unbalanced psycho-physical activity, and unfortunately, as we all know, it does not take long to establish a bad habit. So-called "mental" tricks are more common than purely "physical" tricks, and we are well aware that, when indulged in, they soon become a habit, and that the indulgence of one bad habit tends to the development of others, with a rapid increase in the degree of indulgence.

In this matter of bad habits, and the lack of control which they connote, we must recognize the fact that the human creature cannot be expected to exercise control in the different spheres of his activity in civilization, unless he is in possession of reliable sensory appreciation and of a satisfactory use of the psycho-physical mechanisms involved. People who are lacking in control will be found to be imperfectly co-ordinated, and their sensory appreciation to be unreliable, and no form of discipline or other outside influence can secure that satisfactory standard of psycho-physical functioning without which the individual cannot command a satisfactory standard of control within or without the organism.

Where the human being manifests this lack of control, he needs to be re-educated on a general basis so that reliable sensory appreciation may be restored, together with a satisfactory employment of the psycho-physical mechanisms. The processes of this form of re-education demand that the "means-whereby" to any "end" must be reasoned out, not on a specific but on a general basis, and with the continued use of these processes of reasoning, uncontrolled impulses and "emotional gusts" will gradually cease to dominate, and will ultimately be dominated. The organism will not then be called upon to satisfy those unhealthy cravings which we find associated with unreliable and delusive sensory appreciation (debauched kinæsthesia).

The fact is, the principle of reasoning out on a general basis the *means whereby* we shall command our "ends" simply implies a common-sense procedure. Common sense is a very familiar phrase and we all have our particular conception of what it means. We know many people who will point out that individual opinion can differ as much in regard to the meaning of common sense, as in regard to religious, political, social, and educational matters. We will therefore put our point of view in regard to common sense by giving an instance in which we consider the human creature does not evince common sense. The man who is convinced that he is suffering from digestive and liver disorders, and knows that this has been caused by his indulgence in alcohol, or by excessive eating, and still continues to indulge in either of these habits, despite the depression and suffering which result, and despite the assurance of his medical adviser that moderation will put him on the road to good health once more, cannot be said to act in accordance with common sense.

My reader may say that the man cannot refrain from taking alcohol or from over-eating, and it may be advantageous to consider this man's ability to act in accordance with the dictates of common sense. In the first place, it is clear that he had recognized the fact that he was ill. The fact that he had consulted his medical adviser is proof that the stimulus (or stimuli) in this connexion had reached his consciousness, and no doubt he was quite ready to take the medicine or carry out the form of treatment prescribed, provided that these did not interfere with his habit of indulging in alcohol or in over-eating. But, of course, the desired return to health could not be secured by such an unreasoning procedure. The habit is always the impeding factor and, in this case, the medicine and the treatment were of little importance unless the bad habit of over-indulgence in alcohol, or of excessive feeding, could be eradicated.

This leads us to the consideration of the psycho-physical activities within the organism of which habit, so-called, is a manifestation. In the case of a person who is blessed with a satisfactory standard of psycho-physical co-ordination, moderation will be the rule and excess the exception to that rule. With the person who is badly co-ordinated, the reverse will be the case, in a more or less degree, in one or more spheres, for the habit of excess will gradually become more firmly established with too frequent repetition of the indulgence of the debauched sensory desires connected, in the case given, with eating and drinking, thus making indulgence the rule and not the exception.

In the continuance of our consideration we will trace the cultivation of the alcohol habit, where the subject of our illustration is concerned. That we speak of the cultivation of this habit presupposes a time in the history of the man when he did not make a habit of taking alcohol in such quantities as would cause liver and other internal disorders. The facts concerned with his reasons, however, for beginning to take alcohol to excess at some particular time of his life would not help us very much, even if we could be certain of them. The important point for us to remember is that his sensory appreciation was unreliable and perverted, and his psychophysical organism in an unsatisfactory state of co-ordination, so that he gradually became dominated by that sensory debauchery which results from excessive alcoholic and other indulgence, and by the depressing and enervating conditions which follow. These latter conditions are among the most potent of the stimuli which make for the repetition of the excesses at more and more frequent intervals, this repetition counteracting again for a time the depressing and enervating conditions brought about by the renewed indulgence. Unfortunately, the process is one that "makes the meat it feeds on," so that the degree of sensory debauchery increases rapidly until the functioning of the organism becomes utterly demoralized.

It is almost certain that in the early stages of his alcoholic experiences, the subject was unaware of his lack of satisfactory co-ordination and sensory appreciation. As a matter of fact, it is unlikely that he had ever given consideration to his psycho-physical condition. He had simply taken alcohol occasionally, as he had taken many other things in the way of food and drink, never for a moment meaning that it should become a habit, or even suspecting that he lacked the ability either to continue taking it only occasionally, or to discontinue taking it altogether if he so wished. This reveals the degree to which egotism may be subconsciously developed in the human creature, until it becomes a potent factor in influencing the processes associated with subconscious and unreasoned conclusions, such as the one arrived at by the subject of our illustration in regard to his ability to continue to drink occasionally or to discontinue drinking altogether. If he had consciously attempted to search out the correct premises from which to make his deductions, and if his effort had been attended with success, he would have discovered the unsatisfactory standard of his general functioning, and this would have brought a realization that he must, by some means, make certain that his standard of psycho-physical co-ordination and sensory appreciation was satisfactory, before he allowed himself to entertain even mildly egotistical conclusions regarding his ability to fight his bad habits. If such an analysis of the psycho-physical factors involved had been made, he must have been led to the conclusion that *in the matter of the breaking of habit, the standard of sensory appreciation is the all-important factor.* His increasing desire for alcohol probably came very gradually, as also the corresponding decline in his standard of co-ordination and sensory appreciation. Thus the gratification experienced in satisfying the already abnormal desire would soon dominate psycho-physical processes which otherwise might have been exercised in the field of reasoning and common sense, and he might then have been led to a consideration of the consequences of permitting himself to become a victim of the alcohol habit.

In all such experiences, there comes a time at last when the person concerned is forced to recognize the harmful effects of such a habit, and then very often makes an effort to fight the desire and to eradicate the habit. But too frequently it happens that the effort is a feeble one or that it is made along impossible lines. Some well-meaning friend, for instance, may urge the man to use what is called "will-power" to fight and control his desire, *but the desire is a sensory desire and the processes called "will-power" have in this case long since been dominated by the debauched sensory appreciation associated with this desire,* and therefore his hope of salvation lies in the restoration of his sensory appreciation to that normal condition which we do not find associated with abnormal and unhealthy desire. In a foregoing chapter we have referred to that degenerate state of the organism when the human creature will desire a form of sensory satisfaction through actual pain. In the case of alcoholic excesses, each occasion of indulgence is followed by suffering, often intense suffering, but even this does not act as a deterrent. We must therefore realize the enormous influence of perverted sensory desire on the human creature, and recognize that satisfactory development in the control of his psycho-physical processes is impossible without that reliable sensory appreciation which goes hand in hand with normal sensory desires.

One point more. Fundamental desires and needs must be satisfied; if they are not, serious results must follow sooner or later, and the fact that the attempt to satisfy desires and needs leads many individuals to indulge in abuse and excess does not affect this conclusion. Abuse and excess are always associated with abnormality, and abnormality is due to abnormal conditions in the psycho-physical functioning of the organism, and this applies in the matter of abuse and excess in eating, as well as in drinking and in connexion with any other needs and desires. Abuse or excess is an attempt to satisfy a need or desire, which, originally normal, has become abnormal, and as long as this abnormal desire or need remains, it is useless to deny a man the "means-whereby" to his excesses and abuses. Our energies should instead be applied to attempts to eradicate the abnormal conditions responsible for the excess and abuse, and so to restore the normal psycho-physical functioning of the organism and the reliable sensory appreciation which ensures the maintenance of normality in our desires and needs.

# PART IV
# DISCOVERY

## Chapter One

# THE AUSTRALIAN STORY

From my early youth I took a delight in poetry and it was one of my chief pleasures to study the plays of Shakespeare, reading them aloud and endeavouring to interpret the characters. This led to my becoming interested in elocution and the art of reciting, and now and again I was asked to recite in public. I was sufficiently successful to think of taking up Shakespearean reciting as a career, and worked long and hard at the study of every branch of dramatic expression. After a certain amount of experience as an amateur, I reached the stage when I believed that my work could stand the severer test of being judged from the professional standard, and the criticisms I received justified me in deciding to take up reciting as a profession.

All went well for some years, when I began to have trouble with my throat and vocal cords, and not long after I was told by my friends that when I was reciting my breathing was audible, and that they could hear me (as they put it) "gasping" and "sucking in air" through my mouth. This worried me even more than my actual throat trouble which was then in its early stages, for I had always prided myself on being free from the habit of audibly sucking in breath which is so common with reciters, actors and singers. I therefore sought the advice of doctors and voice trainers in the hope of remedying my faulty breathing and relieving my hoarseness, but in spite of all that they could do in the way of treatment, the gasping and sucking in of breath when I was reciting became more and more exaggerated and the hoarseness recurred at shorter intervals.[1] The treatment I was receiving became less and less effective as time went on, and the trouble gradually increased until, after a few years, I found to my dismay that I had

[1] The medical diagnosis in my case was irritation of the mucous membrane of the throat and nose, and inflammation of the vocal cords which were said to be unduly relaxed. My uvula was very long and at times caused acute attacks of coughing. For this reason two of my medical advisers recommended it should be shortened by a minor operation, but I did not follow this advice. I now have little doubt that I was suffering from what is sometimes called "clergyman's sore throat."

developed a condition of hoarseness which from time to time culmi-
nated in a complete loss of voice. I had experienced a good deal
of ill-health all my life and this had often been a stumbling-block
to me, so that with the additional burden of my recurring hoarseness, I began to doubt the soundness of my vocal organs. The
climax came when I was offered a particularly attractive and important engagement, for by this time I had reached such a stage of
uncertainty about the conditions of my vocal organs that I was
frankly afraid to accept it. I decided to consult my doctor once
more, even though the previous treatment had been disappointing.
After making a fresh examination of my throat, he promised me
that if, during the fortnight before my recital, I abstained from
reciting and used my voice as little as possible and agreed to follow
the treatment he prescribed, my voice by the end of that time would
be normal.

I acted on his advice and accepted the engagement. After a few
days I felt assured that the doctor's promise would be fulfilled, for
I found that by using my voice as little as possible I gradually lost
my hoarseness. When the night of my recital came, I was quite free
from hoarseness, but before I was halfway through my programme,
my voice was in the most distressing condition again, and by the
end of the evening the hoarseness was so acute that I could hardly
speak.

My disappointment was greater than I can express, for it now
seemed to me that I could never look forward to more than a temporary relief, and that I should thus be forced to give up a career
in which I had become deeply interested and believed I could be
successful.

I saw my doctor next day and we talked the matter over, and
at the end of the talk I asked him what he thought we had better do
about it. "We must go on with the treatment," he said. I told him
I could not do that, and when he asked me why, I pointed out to
him that although I had faithfully carried out his instruction not
to use my voice in public during his treatment, the old condition
of hoarseness had returned within an hour after I started to use
my voice again on the night of my recital. "Is it not fair, then," I
asked him, "to conclude that it was *something I was doing that
evening in using my voice that was the cause of the trouble?*" He

thought a moment and said, "Yes, that must be so." "Can you tell me, then," I asked him, *"what it was that I did* that caused the trouble?" He frankly admitted that he could not. "Very well," I replied, "if that is so, I must try and find out for myself."

When I set out on this investigation, I had two facts to go on. I had learned by experience that reciting brought about conditions of hoarseness, and that this hoarseness tended to disappear, as long as I confined the use of my voice to ordinary speaking, and at the same time had medical treatment for my throat and vocal organs. I considered the bearing of these two facts upon my difficulty, and I saw that if ordinary speaking did not cause hoarseness while reciting did, there must be something different between what I did in reciting and what I did in ordinary speaking. If this were so, and I could find out what the difference was, it might help me to get rid of the hoarseness, and at least I could do no harm by making an experiment.

To this end I decided to make use of a mirror and observe the manner of my "doing" both in ordinary speaking and reciting, hoping that this would enable me to distinguish the difference, if any, between them, and it seemed better to begin by watching myself during the simpler act of ordinary speaking, in order to have something to go by when I came to watch myself during the more exacting act of reciting.

Standing before a mirror I first watched myself carefully during the act of ordinary speaking. I repeated the act many times, but saw nothing in my manner of doing it that seemed wrong or unnatural. I then went on to watch myself carefully in the mirror when I recited, and I very soon noticed several things that I had not noticed when I was simply speaking. I was particularly struck by three things that I saw myself doing. I saw that as soon as I started to recite, I tended "to pull back the head," depress the larynx and suck in breath through the mouth in such a way as to produce a gasping sound.

After I had noticed these tendencies I went back and watched myself again during ordinary speaking, and on this occasion I was left in little doubt that the three tendencies I had noticed for the first time when reciting were also present, though in a lesser degree, in my ordinary speaking. They were indeed so slight that I could understand why, on the previous occasions when I had watched myself in ordinary speaking[1] I had altogether failed to notice them. When I discovered this marked difference between what I did in ordinary speaking and what I did in reciting, I realized that here I had a definite fact which might explain many things, and I was encouraged to go on.

I recited again and again in front of the mirror and found that the three tendencies I had already noticed became specially marked when I was reciting passages in which unusual demands were made upon my voice. This served to confirm my early suspicion that there might be some connexion between what I did with myself while reciting and my throat trouble, a not unreasonable supposition, it seemed to me, since what I did in ordinary speaking caused no noticeable harm, while what I did in reciting to meet any unusual demands on my voice brought about an acute condition of hoarseness.

From this I was led to conjecture that if pulling back my head, depressing my larynx and sucking in breath did indeed bring about a strain on my voice, it must constitute a misuse of the parts concerned. I now believed I had found the root of the trouble, for I argued that if my hoarseness arose from the way I used parts of my organism, I should get no further unless I could prevent or change this misuse.

When, however, I came to try to make practical use of this discovery, I found myself in a maze. For where was I to begin? Was it the sucking in of breath that caused the pulling back of the head and the depressing of the larynx? Or was it the pulling back of the head that caused the depressing of the larynx and the sucking in of breath? Or was it the depressing of the larynx that caused the sucking in of breath and the pulling back of the head?

As I was unable to answer these questions, all I could do was to go on patiently experimenting before the mirror. After some months I found that when reciting I could not by direct means prevent the sucking in of breath or the depressing of the larynx,

---

[1] This could hardly have been otherwise, seeing that I then lacked experience in the kind of observation necessary to enable me to detect anything wrong in the way I used myself when speaking.

but that I could to some extent prevent the pulling back of the head. This led me to a discovery which turned out to be of great importance, namely, that when I succeeded in preventing the pulling back of the head, this tended indirectly to check the sucking in of breath and the depressing of the larynx.

The importance of this discovery cannot be overestimated, for through it I was led on to the further discovery of the primary control of the working of all the mechanisms of the human organism, and this marked the first important stage of my investigation.

A further result, which I also noted was that with the prevention of the misuse of these parts I tended to become less hoarse while reciting, and that as I gradually gained experience in this prevention, my liability to hoarseness tended to decrease. What is more, when, after these experiences, my throat was again examined by my medical friends, a considerable improvement was found in the general condition of my larynx and vocal cords.

In this way it was borne in upon me that the changes in *use* that I had been able to bring about by preventing the three harmful tendencies I had detected in myself had produced a marked effect upon the *functioning* of my vocal and respiratory mechanisms.

This conclusion, I now see, marked the second important stage in my investigations, for my practical experience in this specific instance brought me to realize for the first time the close connexion that exists between use and functioning.

My experience up till now had shewn me

(1) that the tendency to put my head back was associated with my throat trouble, and
(2) that I could relieve this trouble to a certain extent merely by preventing myself from putting my head back, since this act of prevention tended to prevent indirectly the depressing of the larynx and the sucking in of breath.

From this I argued that if I put my head definitely forward, I might be able to influence the functioning of my vocal and respiratory mechanisms still further in the right direction, and so eradicate the tendency to hoarseness altogether. I therefore decided as my next step to put my head definitely forward, further forward, in fact, than I felt was the right thing to do.

When I came to try it, however, I found that after I had put my head forward beyond a certain point, I tended to pull it down as well as forward, and, as far as I could see, the effect of this upon my vocal and respiratory organs was much the same as when I pulled my head back and down. For in both acts there was the same depressing of the larynx that was associated with my throat trouble, and by this time I was convinced that this depressing of the larynx must be checked if my voice was ever to become normal. I therefore went on experimenting in the hope of finding some use of the head and neck which was not associated with a depressing of the larynx.

It is impossible to describe here in detail my various experiences during this long period. Suffice it to say that in the course of these experiments I came to notice that any use of my head and neck which was associated with a depressing of the larynx was also associated with a tendency to lift the chest and shorten[1] the stature.

As I look back I realize that this again was a discovery of far-reaching implications, and events proved that it marked a turning-point in my investigations.

This new piece of evidence suggested that the functioning of the organs of speech was influenced by my manner of using the whole torso, and that the pulling of the head back and down was not, as I had presumed, merely a misuse of the specific parts concerned, but one that was inseparably bound up with a misuse of other mechanisms which involved the act of shortening the stature. If this were so, it would clearly be useless to expect such improvement as I needed from merely preventing the wrong use of the head and neck. I realized that I must also prevent those other associated wrong uses which brought about the shortening of the stature.

This led me on to a long series of experiments in some of which

---

[1] Although it would probably be more correct to use the phrases *"increase* the stature," *"decrease* the stature," I have decided to use the phrases "lengthen the stature," "shorten the stature," because the words "lengthen" and "shorten" are those most commonly used in this connexion.

I attempted to prevent the shortening of the stature, in others actually to lengthen it, noting the results in each case. For a time I alternated between these two forms of experiment, and after noting the effect of each upon my voice, I found that the best conditions of my larynx and vocal mechanisms and the least tendency to hoarseness were associated with a *lengthening* of the stature. Unfortunately, I found that when I came to practise, I shortened far more than I lengthened, and when I came to look for an explanation of this, I saw that it was due to my tendency to pull my head down as I tried to put it forward in order to lengthen. After further experimentation I found at last that in order to maintain a lengthening of the stature it was necessary that my head should tend to go upwards, not downwards, when I put it forward; in short, that to lengthen I *must put my head forward and up.*

As is shewn by what follows, this proved to be the primary control of my use in all my activities.

When, however, I came to try to put my head forward and up *while reciting,* I noticed that my old tendency to lift the chest increased, and that with this went a tendency to increase the arch of the spine and thus bring about what I now call a "narrowing of the back." This, I saw, had an adverse effect on the shape and functioning of the torso itself, and I therefore concluded that to maintain a lengthening it was not sufficient to put my head forward and up, but that I must put it forward and up in such a way that I prevented the lifting of the chest and simultaneously brought about a widening of the back.

Having got so far, I considered I should now be justified in attempting to put these findings into practice. To this end I proceeded in my vocal work to try to prevent my old habit of pulling my head back and down and lifting the chest (shortening the stature), and to combine this act of prevention with an attempt to put the head forward and up (lengthening the stature) and widen the back. This was my first attempt to combine "prevention" and "doing" in one activity, and I never for a moment doubted that I should be able to do this, but I found that although I was now able to put the head forward and up and widen the back as acts in themselves, *I could not maintain these conditions in speaking or reciting.*

This made me suspicious that I was not doing what I thought

I was doing, and I decided once more to bring the mirror to my aid. Later on I took into use two additional mirrors, one on each side of the central one, and with their aid I found that my suspicions were justified. For there I saw that at the critical moment when I tried to combine the prevention of shortening with a positive attempt to *maintain a lengthening and speak at the same time,* I did not put my head forward and up as I intended, but actually put it back. Here then was a startling proof that I was doing the opposite of what I believed I was doing and of what I had decided I ought to do.

I break my story here to draw attention to a very curious fact, even though it tells against myself. My reader will remember that in my earlier experiments, when I wished to make certain of what I was doing with myself in the familiar act of reciting, I had derived invaluable help from the use of a mirror. Despite this past experience and the knowledge that I had gained from it, I now set out on an experiment which brought into play a new use of certain parts and involved sensory experiences that were totally unfamiliar, without its even occurring to me that for this purpose I should need the help of the mirror more than ever.

This shews how confident I was, in spite of my past experience, that I should be able to put into practice any idea that I thought desirable. When I found myself unable to do so, I thought that this was merely a personal idiosyncrasy, but my teaching experience of the past thirty-five years and my observation of people with whom I have come into contact in other ways have convinced me that this was not an idiosyncrasy, but that most people would have done the same in similar circumstances. I was indeed suffering from a delusion that is practically universal, the delusion that because we are able to do what we "will to do" in acts that are habitual and involve familiar sensory experiences, we shall be equally successful in doing what we "will to do" in acts which are contrary to our habit and therefore involve sensory experiences that are unfamiliar.

When I realized this, I was much disturbed and I saw that the whole situation would have to be reconsidered. I went back to the beginning again, to my original conclusion that the cause of my throat trouble was to be found in something I was doing myself when I used my voice. I had since discovered both what this "something" was and what I believed I ought to do instead, if my vocal organs were to function properly. But this had not helped me much, for when the time came for me to apply what I had learned to my reciting, and I had tried to do what I ought to do, I had failed. Obviously, then, my next step was to find out at what point in my "doing" I had gone wrong.

There was nothing for it but to persevere, and I practised patiently month after month, as I had been doing hitherto, with varying experiences of success and failure, but without much enlightenment. In time, however, I profited by these experiences, for through them I came to see that any attempt to maintain my lengthening when reciting not only involved on my part the prevention of the wrong use of certain specific parts and the substitution of what I believed to be a better use of these parts, but that this attempt also involved my bringing into play the use of all those parts of the organism required for the activities incident to the act of reciting, such as standing, walking, using the arms or hands for gesture, interpretation, etc.

Observation in the mirror shewed me that when I was standing to recite I was using these other parts in certain wrong ways which synchronized with my wrong way of using my head and neck, larynx, vocal and breathing organs, and which involved a condition of undue muscle tension throughout my organism. I observed that this condition of undue muscle tension affected particularly the use of my legs, feet and toes, my toes being contracted and bent downwards in such a way that my feet were unduly arched, my weight thrown more on to the outside of my feet than it should have been, and my balance interfered with.

On discovering this, I thought back to see if I could account for it, and I recalled an instruction that had been given to me in the past by the late Mr. James Cathcart (at one time a member of Mr. Charles Kean's Company) when I was taking lessons from him in dramatic expression and interpretation. Not being pleased with my way of standing and walking, he would say to me from time to time, "Take hold of the floor with your feet." He would then proceed to shew me what he meant by this, and I did my best to copy him, believing that if I was told what to do to correct something that was wrong, I should be able to do it and all would be well. I persevered and in time believed that my way of standing was now satisfactory, because I thought I was "taking hold of the floor with my feet" as I had seen him do.

The belief is very generally held that if only we are told what to do in order to correct a wrong way of doing something, we can do it, and that if we *feel* we are doing it, all is well. All my experience, however, goes to shew that this belief is a delusion.

On recalling this experience I continued with the aid of mirrors to observe the use of myself more carefully than ever, and came to realize that what I was doing with my legs, feet and toes when standing to recite was exerting a most harmful general influence upon the use of myself throughout my organism. This convinced me that the use of these parts involved an abnormal amount of muscle tension and was indirectly associated with my throat trouble, and I was strengthened in this conviction when I reminded myself that my teacher had found it necessary in the past to try and improve my way of standing in order to get better results in my reciting. It gradually dawned upon me that the wrong way I was using myself when I thought I was "taking hold of the floor with my feet" was the same wrong way I was using myself when in reciting I pulled my head back, depressed my larynx, etc., and that this wrong way of using myself constituted a combined wrong use of the whole of my physical-mental mechanisms. I then realized that this was the use which I habitually brought into play for all my activities, that it was what I may call the "habitual use" of myself, and that my desire to recite, like any other stimulus to activity, would inevitably cause this habitual wrong use to come into play and dominate any attempt I might be making to employ a better use of myself in reciting.

The influence of this wrong use was bound to be strong because of its being habitual, but in my case it was greatly strengthened because during the past years I had undoubtedly been cultivating it through my efforts to carry out my teacher's instructions to "take hold of the floor with my feet" when I recited. The influence of this *cultivated* habitual use, therefore, acted as an almost irresistible stimulus to me to use myself in the wrong way I was accustomed to; this stimulus to general wrong use was far stronger than the stimulus of my desire to employ the new use of my head and neck, and I now saw that it was this influence which led me, as soon as I stood up to recite, to put my head in the opposite direction to that which I desired. I now had proof of one thing at least, that all my efforts up till now to improve the use of myself in reciting had been misdirected.

It is important to remember that the use of a specific part in any activity is closely associated with the use of other parts of the organism, and that the influence exerted by the various parts one upon another is continuously changing in accordance with the manner of use of these parts. If a part directly employed in the activity is being used in a comparatively new way which is still unfamiliar, the stimulus to use this part in the new way is weak in comparison with the stimulus to use the other parts of the organism, which are being indirectly employed in the activity, in the old habitual way.

In the present case, an attempt was being made to bring about an unfamiliar use of the head and neck for the purpose of reciting. The stimulus to employ the new use of the head and neck was therefore bound to be weak as compared with the stimulus to employ the wrong habitual use of the feet and legs which had become familiar through being cultivated in the act of reciting.

Herein lies the difficulty in making changes from unsatisfactory to satisfactory conditions of use and functioning, and my teaching experience has taught me that when a wrong habitual use has been cultivated in a person for whatever purpose, its influence in the early stages of the lessons is practically irresistible.

This led me to a long consideration of the whole question of the direction[1] of the use of myself. "What is this direction," I asked myself, "upon which I have been depending?" I had to admit that I had never thought out how I directed the use of myself, but that I used myself habitually in the way that *felt natural* to me. In other words, I, like everyone else, depending upon "feeling" for the direction of my use. Judging, however, from the results of my experiments, this method of direction had led me into error (as,

[1] When I employ the words "direction" and "directed" with "use" in such phrases as "direction of my use" and "I directed the use," etc., I wish to indicate the process involved in projecting messages from the brain to the mechanisms and in conducting the energy necessary to the use of these mechanisms.

for instance, when I put my head back when I intended to put it forward and up), proving that the "feeling" associated with this direction of my use was untrustworthy.

This indeed was a blow. If ever anyone was in an impasse, it was I. For here I was, faced with the fact that my feeling, the only guide I had to depend upon for the direction of my use, was untrustworthy. At the time I believed that this was peculiar to myself, and that my case was exceptional because of the continuous ill-health I had experienced for as long as I could remember, but as soon as I tested other people to see whether they were using themselves in the way they thought they were, I found that the feeling by which they directed the use of themselves was also untrustworthy, indeed, that the only difference in this regard between them and myself was one of degree. Discouraged as I was, however, I refused to believe that the problem was hopeless. I began to see that my findings up till now implied the possibility of the opening up of an entirely new field of enquiry, and I was obsessed with the desire to explore it. "Surely," I argued, "if it is possible for feeling to become untrustworthy as a means of direction, it should also be possible to make it trustworthy again."

The idea of the wonderful potentialities of man had been a source of inspiration to me ever since I had come to know Shakespeare's great word picture:

*What a piece of work is a man! how noble in reason! how infinite in faculty! in form and moving how express and admirable! in action how like an angel! in apprehension how like a god! the beauty of the world! the paragon of animals!*

But these words seemed to me now to be contradicted by what I had discovered in myself and others. For what could be less "noble in reason," less "infinite in faculty," than that man, despite his potentialities, should have fallen into such error in the use of himself, and in this way brought about such a lowering in his standard of functioning that in everything he attempts to accomplish, these harmful conditions tend to become more and more exaggerated? In consequence, how many people are there today of whom it may be said, as regards their use of themselves, "in form and moving how express and admirable"? Can we any longer consider man in this regard "the paragon of animals"?

I can remember at this period discussing with my father the errors in use which I had noticed both in myself and in others, and contending that in this respect there was no difference between us and the dog or cat. When he asked me why, I replied, "Because we do not *know* how we use ourselves any more than the dog or cat *knows*." By this I meant that man's direction of his use, through being based upon feeling, was as unreasoned and instinctive as that of the animal.[1] I refer to this conversation as shewing that I had already realized that in our present state of civilization which calls for continuous and rapid adaptation to a quickly changing environment, the unreasoned, instinctive direction of use such as meets the needs of the cat or dog was no longer sufficient to meet human needs. I had proved in my own case and in that of others that instinctive control and direction of use had become so unsatisfactory, and the associated feeling so untrustworthy as a guide, that it could lead us to do the very opposite of what we wished to do or thought we were doing. If, then, as I suspected, this untrust-

---

[1] It may be contended that the athlete who successfully performs a complicated feat does consciously control his movements. It is true, of course, that in a great many cases he is able by practice on the "trial and error" plan to acquire an automatic proficiency in performing the specific movements necessary for this feat, but this does not in any way prove that he is controlling these movements consciously. And even in those rare instances where the athlete consciously controls and coördinates certain specific movements, it still cannot be said that he consciously controls the use of himself as a whole in his performance. For it is safe to conclude that he does not *know* what use of his mechanisms as a whole is the best possible for making the specific movements he desires, so that should anything happen, as it often does, to cause a change in the familiar habitual use of his mechanisms, his proficiency in making these specific movements will also be interfered with. Practical experience shews that once he has lost this original standard of proficiency, he cannot easily regain it, and this is not surprising seeing that he lacks the knowledge of how to direct the general use of himself which alone would enable him to restore the familiar use of his mechanisms which gave him his proficiency. (In this connexion, many cases have been known of people who, having purposely imitated the peculiarities of a stutterer, have themselves developed the habit of stuttering, and in spite of all their efforts have failed to regain their original standard of proficiency in speaking.)

Because he lacks this knowledge, the athlete, like the animal, has to depend upon his feeling for the direction of the working of his mechanisms, and as that feeling has become more or less untrustworthy in the majority of athletes (a fact that can be demonstrated), the mechanisms which he employs for his activities are bound to be misdirected. Such direction, being as unreasoned as that of the animal, cannot be compared with that conscious reasoned direction which is associated with a primary control of the mechanisms of the self as a working unity.

worthiness of feeling was a product of civilized life, it would tend, as time went on, to become more and more a universal menace, in which case a knowledge of the means whereby trustworthiness could be restored to feeling would be invaluable. I saw that the search for this knowledge would open out an entirely new field of exploration and one that promised more than any that I had yet heard of, and I began to reconsider my own difficulties in the light of this new fact.

Certain points impressed themselves particularly upon me:

(1) that the pulling of my head back and down, when I *felt* that I was putting it forward and up, was proof that the use of the specific parts concerned was being misdirected, and that this misdirection was associated with untrustworthy feeling;

(2) that this misdirection was instinctive, and, together with the associated untrustworthy feeling, was part and parcel of my habitual use of myself;

(3) that this instinctive misdirection leading to wrong habitual use of myself, including most noticeably the wrong use of my head and neck, *came into play as the result of a decision to use my voice; this misdirection, in other words, was my instinctive response (reaction) to the stimulus to use my voice.*

When I came to consider the significance of this last point, it occurred to me that if, when the stimulus came to me to use my voice, I could inhibit the misdirection associated with the wrong habitual use of my head and neck, I should be stopping off at its source my unsatisfactory reaction to the idea of reciting, which expressed itself in pulling back the head, depressing the larynx, and sucking in breath. Once this misdirection was inhibited, my next step would be to discover what direction would be necessary to ensure a new and improved use of the head and neck, and, indirectly, of the larynx and breathing and other mechanisms, for I believed that such direction, when put into practice, would ensure a satisfactory instead of an unsatisfactory reaction to the stimulus to use my voice.

In the work that followed I came to see that to get a direction of my use which would *ensure* this satisfactory reaction, I must cease to rely upon the feeling associated with my instinctive direction, and in its place employ my reasoning processes, in order

(1) to analyse the conditions of use present;
(2) to select (reason out) the means whereby a more satisfactory use could be brought about;
(3) to project *consciously* the directions required for putting these means into effect.

In short, I concluded that if I were ever able to react satisfactorily to the stimulus to use my voice, I must replace my old instinctive (unreasoned) direction of myself by a new conscious (reasoned) direction.

The idea of taking the control of the use of the mechanisms of the human creature from the instinctive on to the conscious plane has already been justified by the results which have been obtained by applying it in practice, but it may be many years before its true significance as a factor in human development is fully recognized.

I set out to put this idea into practice, but I was at once brought up short by a series of startling and unexpected experiences. Like most people, I had believed up to this moment that if I thought out carefully how to improve my way of performing a certain act, I should be guided by my reasoning rather than by my feeling when it came to putting this thought into action, and that my "mind" was the superior and more effective directing agent. But the fallacy of this became apparent to me as soon as I attempted to employ conscious direction for the purpose of correcting some wrong use of myself which was habitual and therefore *felt right* to me. In actual practice I found that there was no clear dividing line between my unreasoned and my reasoned direction of myself, and that I was quite unable to prevent the two from overlapping. I was successful in employing my reasoning up to the point of projecting the directions which, after analysing the conditions of use present, I had decided were required for the new and improved use, and all went well as long as I did not attempt to carry these directions out for the purpose of speaking. For instance, as soon as any stimulus reached me to use my voice, and I tried in response to *do* the new thing which my conscious direction should bring about (such as putting the head forward and up), and *speak at the same time,* I found I immediately reverted to all my old wrong habits of use (such as putting my head back, etc.). There was no question about this. I could see it actually happening in the mirror. This was clear proof that at the critical moment when I attempted to gain my end by means which were contrary to those associated with my old habits of use, my instinctive direction dominated my reasoning direction. It dominated my will to do what I had decided was the right thing to do, and although I was trying (as we understand "trying") to do it. Over and over again I had the experience that immediately the stimulus to speak came to me, I invariably responded by doing something according to my old habitual use associated with the act of speaking.

After many disappointing experiences of this kind I decided to give up any attempt for the present to "do" anything to gain my end, and I came to see at last that if I was ever to be able to change my habitual use and dominate my instinctive direction, *it would be necessary for me to make the experience of receiving the stimulus to speak and of refusing to do anything immediately in response.* For I saw that an immediate response was the result of a decision on my part to do something *at once,* to go directly for a certain end, and by acting quickly on this decision I did not give myself the opportunity to project as many times as was necessary the new directions which I had reasoned out were the best means whereby I could attain that end. This meant that the old instinctive direction which, associated with untrustworthy feeling, had been the controlling factor up to that moment in the building up of my wrong habitual use, still controlled the *manner* of my response, with the inevitable result that my old wrong habitual use was again brought into play.

I therefore decided to confine my work to giving myself the directions for the new "means-whereby,"[1] instead of actually trying to "do" them or to relate them to the "end" of speaking. I would give the new directions in front of the mirror for long periods together, for successive days and weeks and sometimes even months,

[1] The phrase "means-whereby" is used to indicate the reasoned means to the gaining of an end. These means included the inhibition of the habitual use of the mechanisms of the organism, and the conscious projection of new directions necessary to the performance of the different acts involved in a new and more satisfactory use of these mechanisms.

without attempting to "do" them, and the experience I gained in giving these directions proved of great value when the time came for me to consider how to put them into practice.

This experience taught me

(1) that before attempting to "do" even the first part of the new "means-whereby" which I had decided to employ in order to gain my end (i.e., vocal use and reciting), I must give the directions preparatory to the doing of this first part very many times;

(2) that I must *continue* to give the directions preparatory to the doing of the first part while I gave the directions preparatory to the doing of the second part;

(3) that I must *continue* to give the directions preparatory to the doing of the first and second parts while I gave the directions preparatory to the doing of the third part; and so on for the doing of the fourth and other parts as required.

Lastly, I discovered that after I had become familiar with the combined process of giving the directions for the new "means-whereby" in their sequence and of employing the various corresponding mechanisms in order to bring about the new use, I must continue this process in my practice for a considerable time before actually attempting to employ the new "means-whereby" for the purpose of speaking.

The process I have just described is an example of what Professor John Dewey has called "thinking in activity," and anyone who carries it out faithfully while trying to gain an end will find that he is acquiring a new experience in what he calls "thinking." My daily teaching experience shews me that in working for a given end, we can all project one direction, but to continue to give this direction as we project the second, and to continue to give these two while we add a third, and to continue to keep the three directions going as we proceed to gain the end, has proved to be the *pons asinorum* of every pupil I have so far known.[1]

The time came when I believed I had practised the "means-

---

[1] The phrase "all together, one after the other" expresses the idea of combined activity I wish to convey here.

whereby" long enough, and I started to try and employ them for the purpose of speaking, but to my dismay I found that I failed far more often than I succeeded. The further I went with these attempts, the more perplexing the situation became, for I was certainly attempting to inhibit my habitual response to the stimulus to speak, and I had certainly given the new directions over and over again. At least, this is what I had intended to do and thought I had done, so that, as far as I could then see, I should have been able to employ the new "means-whereby" for the gaining of my end with some degree of confidence. The fact remained that I failed more often than not, and nothing was more certain than that I must go back and reconsider my premises.

This reconsideration shewed me more clearly than ever that the occasions when I failed were those on which I was unable to prevent the dominance of my wrong habitual use, as I attempted to employ the new "means-whereby" with the idea of gaining my end and speaking. I also saw (and this was of the utmost importance) that, in spite of all my preliminary work, the instinctive direction associated with my habitual use still dominated my conscious reasoning direction. So confident was I, however, that the new means I had chosen were right for my purpose, that I decided I must look elsewhere for the cause of my unsatisfactory results. In time I began to doubt whether perhaps my failures were not due to some shortcoming in myself, and that I personally was unable to do a thing with satisfactory "means-whereby" when someone else might have been successful. I looked all round for any other possible causes of failure, and after a long period of investigation I came to the conclusion that it was necessary for me to seek some concrete proof whether, at the critical moment when I attempted to gain my end and speak, I was really continuing to project the directions in their proper sequence for the employment of the new and more satisfactory use, as I thought I was, or whether I was reverting to the instinctive misdirection of my old habitual use which had been associated with all my throat trouble. By careful experimentation I discovered that I gave my directions for the new use in their sequence right up to the point when I tried to gain my end and speak, but that, at the critical moment when persistence in giving the new directions would have brought success, I reverted instead to the misdirection associated with my old wrong habitual use. This was concrete proof that I was not continuing to project my directions for the new use for the purpose of speaking, as I thought I was, but that my reaction to the stimulus to speak was still my instinctive reaction through my habitual use. Clearly, to "feel" or think I had inhibited the old instinctive reaction was no proof that I had really done so, and I must find some way of "knowing."

I had already noticed that on the occasions when I failed, the instinctive misdirection associated with my old habitual use always dominated my reasoning direction for the new use, and I gradually came to see that this could hardly be otherwise. Ever since the beginning of man's growth and development the only form of direction of the use of himself of which he has had any experience has been instinctive direction, which might in this sense be called a racial inheritance. Was it then to be wondered at that in my case the influence of this inherited instinctive direction associated with my old habitual use had rendered futile most of my efforts to employ a conscious, reasoning direction for a new use, especially when the use of myself which was associated with instinctive direction had become so familiar that it was now part and parcel of me, and so *felt right and natural?* In trying to employ a conscious, reasoning direction to bring about a new use, I was therefore combating in myself not only that racial tendency which causes us all at critical moments to revert to instinctive direction and so to the familiar use of ourselves that feels right, but also a racial inexperience in projecting conscious directions at all, and particularly conscious directions in sequence.

As the reader knows, I had recognized much earlier that I ought not to trust to my feeling for the direction of my use, but I had never fully realized all that this implied, namely, that the sensory experience associated with the new use would be so unfamiliar and therefore "feel" so unnatural and wrong that I, like everyone else, with my ingrained habit of judging whether experiences of use were "right" or not by the way they *felt,* would almost inevitably balk at employing the new use. Obviously, any new use must feel different from the old, and if the old use felt right, the new use was bound to feel wrong. I now had to face the fact that in all my attempts during these past months I had been trying to employ a new use of myself which was bound to feel wrong, at the same time trusting to my feeling of what was right to tell me whether I was employing it or not. This meant that all my efforts up till now had resolved themselves into an attempt to employ a reasoning direction of my use at the moment of speaking, while for the purpose of this attempt I was actually bringing into play my old habitual use and so reverting to my instinctive misdirection. Small wonder that this attempt had proved futile!

Faced with this, I now saw that if I was ever to succeed in making the changes in use I desired, I must subject the processes directing my use to a new experience, the experience, that is, of being dominated by reasoning instead of by feeling, particularly at the critical moment when the giving of directions merged into "doing" for the gaining of the end I had decided upon. This meant that I must be prepared to carry on with any procedure I had reasoned out as best for my purpose, even though that procedure might *feel wrong*. In other words, my trust in my reasoning processes to bring me safely to my "end" must be a genuine trust, not a half-trust needing the assurance of *feeling right* as well. I must at all costs work out some plan by which to obtain concrete proof that my instinctive reaction to the stimulus to gain my end *remained inhibited*, while I projected in their sequence the directions for the employment of the new use at the critical moment of gaining that end.

After making many attempts to solve this problem and gaining experience which proved to be of great value and interest to me, I finally adopted the following plan.[1]

(1) inhibit any immediate response to the stimulus to speak the sentence.

(2) project in their sequence the directions for the primary control which I had reasoned out as being best for the purpose of bringing about the new and improved use of myself in speaking, and

(3) continue to project these directions until I believed I was sufficiently *au fait* with them to employ them for the purpose of gaining my end and speaking the sentence.

[1] This plan, though simple in theory, has proved difficult for most pupils to put into practice.

At this moment, the moment that had always proved critical for me because it was then that I tended to revert to my wrong habitual use, I would change my usual procedure and

(4) *while still continuing to project the directions for the new use* I would stop and consciously reconsider my first decision, and ask myself "Shall I after all go on to gain the end I have decided upon and speak the sentence? Or shall I not? Or shall I go on to gain some other end altogether?" —*and then and there make a fresh decision,*

(5) either

not to gain my original end, in which case *I would continue to project the directions for maintaining the new use* and not go on to speak the sentence;

or

to change my end and do something different, say, lift my hand instead of speaking the sentence, in which case *I would continue to project the directions for maintaining the new use* to carry out this last decision and lift my hand;

or

to go on after all and gain my original end, in which case *I would continue to project the directions for maintaining the new use* to speak the sentence.

It will be seen that under this new plan the change in procedure came at the critical moment when hitherto, in going on to gain my end, I had so often reverted to instinctive misdirection and my wrong habitual use. I reasoned that if I stopped at that moment and then, *without ceasing to project the directions for the new use,* decided afresh to what end the new use should be employed, I should by this procedure be subjecting my instinctive processes of direction to an experience contrary to any experience in which they had hitherto been drilled. Up to that time the stimulus of a decision to gain a certain end had always resulted in the same habitual activity, involving the projection of the instinctive directions for the use which I habitually employed for the gaining of that end. By this new procedure, *as long as the reasoned directions for the bringing about of new conditions of use were consciously maintained,* the stimulus of a decision to gain a certain end would result in an activity differing from the old habitual activity, in that the old activity could not be controlled outside the gaining of a given end, whereas the new activity could be controlled for the gaining of any end that was consciously desired.

I would point out that this procedure is contrary, not only to any procedure in which our individual instinctive direction has been drilled, but contrary also to that in which man's instinctive processes have been drilled continuously all through his evolutionary experience.

When I came to work on this plan, I found that this reasoning was borne out by experience. For by actually deciding, in the majority of cases, to maintain my new conditions of use either to gain some end other than the one originally decided upon, or simply to refuse to gain the original end, I obtained at last the concrete proof I was looking for, namely, that my instinctive response to the stimulus to gain my original end was not only inhibited at the start, *but remained inhibited right through, whilst my directions for the new use were being projected.* And the experience I gained in maintaining the new manner of use while going on to gain some other end or refusing to gain my original end, helped me to maintain the new use on those occasions when I decided at the critical moment to go on after all and gain my original end and speak the sentence. This was further proof that I was becoming able to defeat any influence of that habitual wrong use in speaking to which my original decision to "speak the sentence" had been the stimulus, and that my conscious, reasoning direction was at last dominating the unreasoning, instinctive direction associated with an unsatisfactory habitual use of myself.

After I had worked on this plan for a considerable time, I became free from my tendency to revert to my wrong habitual use in reciting, and the marked effect of this upon my functioning convinced me that I was at last on the right track, for once free from this tendency, I also became free from the throat and vocal trouble and from the respiratory and nasal difficulties with which I had been beset from birth.

*Chapter Two*

# LESSONS LEARNED FROM IT

I must admit that when I began my investigation, I, in common with most people, conceived of "body" and "mind" as separate parts of the same organism, and consequently believed that human ills, difficulties and shortcomings could be classified as either "mental" or "physical" and dealt with on specifically "mental" or specifically "physical" lines. My practical experiences, however, led me to abandon this point of view and readers of my books will be aware that the technique described in them is based on the opposite conception, namely, that it is *impossible* to separate "mental" and "physical" processes in any form of human activity.

This change in my conception of the human organism has not come about as the outcome of mere theorizing on my part. It has been forced upon me by the experiences which I have gained through my investigations in a new field of practical experimentation upon the living human being.

The letters I receive from my readers shew that a large majority of those who accept the theory of the unity of mental and physical processes in human activity, find difficulty in understanding what the practical working of this theory of unity implies. This difficulty is always coming up in my teaching, but it is possible during a course of lessons to demonstrate to the pupil how the mental and physical work together in the use of the self[1] in all activity. Repeated demonstration of this kind brings conviction, but since the number of pupils one can take, even in a large teaching practice, is naturally limited, the opportunities for giving this demonstration are comparatively few, and I have therefore decided to start at the beginning and relate the history of the investigations which gradually led to the evolution of my technique. I have given as fully as

[1] I wish to make it clear that when I employ the word "use," it is not in that limited sense of the use of any specific part, as, for instance, when we speak of the use of an arm or the use of a leg, but in a much wider and more comprehensive sense applying to the working of the organism in general. For I recognize that the use of any specific part such as the arm or leg involves of necessity bringing into action the different psycho-physical mechanisms of the organism, this concerted activity bringing about the use of the specific part.

161

possible the actual details of experiments I made, telling what I observed and experienced during the process, as I believed that by so doing I should be giving my readers the opportunity to see for themselves the train of events which finally convinced me

(1)  that the so-called "mental" and "physical" are not separate entities;

(2)  that for this reason human ills and shortcomings cannot be classified as "mental" or "physical" and dealt with specifically as such, but that all training, whether it be educative or otherwise, i.e., whether its object be the prevention[1] or elimination of defect, error or disease, must be based upon the indivisible unity of the human organism.

If any reader doubts this, I would ask him if he can furnish any proof that the process involved in the act, say, of lifting an arm, or of walking, talking, going to sleep, starting out to learn something, thinking out a problem, making a decision, giving or withholding consent to a request or wish, or of satisfying a need or sudden impulse, is purely "mental" or purely "physical."

Another source of misunderstanding has arisen through my choice of words for which I have often been criticized. While I do not hold a brief for myself in this regard, I have persistently avoided using words which are labels for ideas and "systems" which I am convinced are fundamentally unsound, and I am able to state that when reasons for such criticism have been given to me, I have always found in my critics a tendency to read into other people's words meanings which fitted in with a particular construction that

---

[1] I use the word "prevention" (and this applies equally to "cure") not because I consider it adequate or wholly suitable for my purpose, but because I cannot find another to take its place. "Prevention" in its fullest sense implies the existence of satisfactory conditions which can be prevented from changing for the worse. In this sense prevention is not possible in practice today, since the conditions now present in the civilized human creature are such that it would be difficult to find anyone who is entirely free from manifestations of wrong use and functioning. When, therefore, I use the terms "prevention" and "cure," I use them in a relative sense only, including under "preventive" measures all attempts to prevent faulty use and functioning of the organism generally as a means of preventing defect, disorder and disease, and under "curative" measures those methods in which the influence of faulty use upon functioning is ignored when dealing with defects, disorder and disease.

they were accustomed to put upon them, and I suggest that the habit and the misunderstanding are closely connected. If the reader will remember that the subject of my study has been, and is, the living psycho-physical organism, which is the sum of a complex of unified processes, he will understand why I refrain as far as is possible from using such terms as "postures," "mental states," "psychological complexes," "body mechanics," "subconscious," or any of the thousand and one labelled concepts, which have, like barnacles, become attached to the complicated idea we have of ourselves owing to the kind of education to which we have been subjected. Instead I prefer to call the psycho-physical organism simply "the self," and to write of it as something "in use," which "functions" and which "reacts." My conception of the human organism or of the self is thus very simple, but can be made difficult by needless complication resulting from the preconceived ideas which readers bring to it.

The question of the nature of use in its relation to functioning and reaction in our daily activities presents a problem requiring solution, and it will be found that the attitude of most people, with very few exceptions, is that Nature makes provision for us in this respect. How often have I been asked, "Why should our use of ourselves go wrong? What is the cause?" and so on.

It is true that Nature has provided us all with the potentiality for the reasoning out of means for preventing wrong use of the self, but we have not developed any preventive measures to this end because we have assumed, quite erroneously, that our manner of use of ourselves cannot go wrong or fail us.

But now that it can be demonstrated that the influence of the manner in which we use ourselves is operating continuously either for or against us every moment of our lives, it is unreasonable to cling to this assumption. A good manner of use of the self exerts an influence for good upon general functioning which is not only continuous, but also grows stronger as time goes on, becoming, that is, a *constant* influence tending always to raise the standard of functioning and improve the manner of reaction. A bad manner of use, on the other hand, continuously exerts an influence for ill tending to lower the standard of general functioning, thus becoming a *constant* influence tending always to interfere with every functional activity arising from our response to stimuli from within and without the self, and harmfully affecting the manner of every reaction.

In estimating the extent of this influence of use upon function-ing and reaction, the vital point to consider is whether it is spas-modic or constant. If by chance it is spasmodic, it will have a com-paratively slight effect upon the nature of the functioning, but if, as is usually the case, it is constant, its effect upon functioning will tend as time goes on to grow stronger and stronger.

We all know that constant attention to what we are doing in the daily round of life makes for success, that constant energizing in a given direction is the most effective way to produce a given result, that constant application to a given task by a slow dull per-son can bring success where a quick brilliant person who indulges in spasmodic application will fail, that constant dripping of water will wear away stone, that constant pressure on parts of the human body produces irritation and pain, that constant repetition of a sound at a given interval will drive men mad, indeed, has actually been employed for that purpose, and that constant indulgence in bad habits leads sooner or later to irritation, undue excitement, de-pression, demoralization and even insanity.

The kind of *constant influence,* therefore, which our manner of use exerts upon functioning, is of the utmost importance. If it is one that tends to raise the standard of general functioning, it will be a constant influence for good, but if it is one that tends to lower this standard, then it will be a constant influence for ill. *Habit, in-deed, may be defined as the manifestation of a constant.*

For this reason we should know and be able to employ the means whereby we can establish a good manner of use as a con-stant. When I was experimenting with various ways of using myself in the attempt to improve the functioning of my vocal organs, I discovered that a certain use of the head in relation to the neck, and of the head and neck in relation to the torso and the other parts of the organism, if consciously and continuously em-ployed, ensures, as was shown in my own case, the establishment of a manner of use of the self *as a whole* which provides the best conditions for raising the standard of the functioning of the various mechanisms, organs and systems. I found that in practice this use of the parts, beginning with the use of the head in relation to the neck, constituted a primary control of the mechanisms *as a whole,* involving control *in process* right through the organism, and that when I interfered with the employment of the primary control of my manner of use, this was always associated with a lowering of the standard of my general functioning. This brought me to realize that I had found a way by which we can judge whether the influence of our manner of use is affecting our general functioning adversely or otherwise, the criterion being whether or not this manner of use is interfering with the correct[1] employment of the primary control.

Unfortunately, the great majority of civilized people have come to use themselves in such a way that in everything they are doing they are constantly interfering in a greater or lesser degree with the correct employment of the primary control of their use, and this interference is an influence constantly operating against them, tending always to lower the standard of functioning within themselves and to limit or affect adversely their achievements in the outside world.

This adverse influence will still be operative even in the case of patients who are undergoing medical, surgical, or any other form of treatment for the "cure" or alleviation of some specific trouble, for it will tend constantly to lower the standard of their general functioning, not only *during* treatment but also *after* it is finished. And this will be so, no matter how successful as a specific "cure" the treatment may be. This applies in all fields of man's activity and also to pupils being taught under any educational method. Whether they are being instructed in a school subject such as mathematics, French, etc., being coached for games or athletics, or being taught the specific technique of some art or craft, the adverse influence of any interference with the correct employment of the primary control of their use will tend constantly to lower the standard of their functioning and the quality of their output.

When, on the other hand, a person's manner of use is such that there is no interference with the correct employment of the primary control, it means that an influence is constantly operating in his favour, tending always to raise the standard of functioning within the self, both in outside activity and during sleep.

[1] When in my writings the terms "correct," "proper," "good," "bad," "satisfactory" are used in connexion with such phrases as "the employment of the primary control" or "the manner of use" it must be understood that they indicate conditions of psycho-physical functioning which are the best for the working of the organism as a whole.

Obviously, in all "doing" there is a comparison of what is to be done and how to do it. Whether we react to this conception by giving consent to do the act, or by withholding that consent, the nature of our reaction is determined by our habitual manner of use of ourselves in which we depend upon feeling for guidance.

It is well known that different people will get a different conception from the same word, spoken or written, and from the same gesture, showing that conception is dependent upon the nature of the impressions taken through the sensory mechanisms which control the functioning of the cells (receptors and conductors) of the eyes and ears, etc. The conception likewise of what is happening within ourselves is dependent upon impressions which come to us through the sense of feeling (sensory appreciation) upon which we mostly rely for guidance in carrying out our daily activities. When our sensory appreciation is deceptive, as is the case more or less with every one today, the impressions we get through it are deceptive also. The extent of this deception depends largely upon the extent to which our manner of use has been put wrong and the nature and degree of the faulty guidance of deceptive feeling. When a certain degree of misuse has been reached, the deceptiveness of these impressions reaches a point where they can mislead us into believing that *we are doing something with some part of ourselves when actually we can be proved to be doing something quite different.* This is equally true of things we believe we think, which more often than not are things we feel.

Here then we have a vicious circle. Directly we get a conception of doing something, we react according to our habitual misuse of ourselves, the functioning of some one part or other is thereby impaired and, as the organism works as a whole, this means that all parts will be more or less affected.

In working out my own problem, I was immediately caught in this vicious circle, for my habitual reaction to any conception of "doing" fitted in with my own peculiarities of misuse and faulty functioning, and with the deceptiveness of sensory appreciation that went with these. As soon, therefore, as I tried to change my reaction *directly,* I found that these impeding influences stood in my way, and there was no escape from the vicious circle.

# APPENDIXES

# THREE PREFACES TO BOOKS BY ALEXANDER

### by John Dewey

## I

Many persons have pointed out the strain which has come upon human nature in the change from a state of animal savagery to present civilization. No one, it seems to me, has grasped the meaning, dangers and possibilities of this change more lucidly and completely than Mr. Alexander. His account of the crises which have ensued upon this evolution is a contribution to a better understanding of every phase of contemporary life. His interpretation centres primarily about the crisis in the physical and moral health of the individual produced by the conflict between the functions of the brain and the nervous system on one side and the functions of digestion, circulation, respiration and the muscular system on the other; but there is no aspect of the maladjustments of modern life which does not receive illumination.

Frank acknowledgment of this internecine warfare in the very heart of our civilization is not agreeable. For this reason it is rarely faced in its entirety. We prefer to deal with its incidents and episodes as if they were isolated accidents and could be overcome one by one in isolation. Those who have seen the conflict have almost always proposed as a remedy either a return to nature, a relapse to the simple life, or else flight to some mystic obscurity. Mr. Alexander exposes the fundamental error in the empirical and palliative methods. When the organs through which any structure, be it physiological, mental or social, are out of balance, when they are unco-ordinated, specific and limited attempts at a cure only exercise the already disordered mechanism. In "improving" one organic structure, they produce a compensatory maladjustment, usually more subtle and more difficult to deal with, somewhere else. The ingeniously inclined will have little difficulty in paralleling Mr.

Alexander's criticism of "physical culture methods" within any field of our economic and political life.

In his criticism of return or relapse to the simpler conditions from which civilised man has departed Mr. Alexander's philosophy appears in its essential features. All such attempts represent an attempt at solution through abdication of intelligence. They all argue, in effect, that since the varied evils have come through development of conscious intelligence, the remedy is to let intelligence sleep, while the pre-intelligent forces, out of which it developed, do their work. The pitfalls into which references to the unconscious and subconscious usually fall have no existence in Mr. Alexander's treatment. He gives these terms a definite and real meaning. They express reliance upon the primitive mind of sense, of unreflection, as against reliance upon *reflective* mind. Mr. Alexander sees the remedy not in a futile abdication of intelligence in order that lower forces may work, but in carrying the power of intelligence further, in making its function one of positive and constructive control. As a layman, I am incompetent to pass judgment upon the particular technique through which he would bring about a control of intelligence over the bodily organism so as not merely to cure but to prevent the present multitudinous maladies of adjustment. But he does not stop with a pious recommendation of such conscious control; he possesses and offers a definite method for its realization, and even a layman can testify, as I am glad to do, to the efficacy of its working in concrete cases.

It did not remain for the author of these pages to eulogise self-mastery or self-control. But these eulogies have too frequently remained in the hortatory and moralistic state. Mr. Alexander has developed a definite procedure, based upon a scientific knowledge of the organism. Popular fear of anything sounding like materialism has put a heavy burden upon humanity. Men are afraid, without even being aware of their fear, to recognise the most wonderful of all the structures of the vast universe—the human body. They have been led to think that a serious notice and regard would somehow involve disloyalty to man's higher life. The discussions of Mr. Alexander breathe reverence for this wonderful instrument of our life, life mental and moral as well as that life which somewhat meaninglessly we call bodily. When such a religious attitude toward the body becomes more general, we shall have an atmosphere favorable to securing the conscious control which is urged.

In the larger sense of education, this whole book is concerned with education. But the writer of these lines was naturally especially attracted to the passages in which Mr. Alexander touches on the problems of education in the narrower sense. The meaning of his principles comes out nowhere better than in his criticisms of repressive schools on one hand and schools of "free expression" on the other. He is aware of the perversions and distortions that spring from that unnatural suppression of childhood which too frequently passes for school training. But he is equally aware that the remedy is not to be sought through a blind reaction in abolition of all control except such as the moment's whim or the accident of environment may provide. One gathers that in this country, Mr. Alexander has made the acquaintance of an extremely rare type of "self-expressive" school, but all interested in educational reform may well remember that freedom of physical action and free expression of emotion are means, not ends, and that as means they are justified only in so far as they are used as conditions for developing power of intelligence. The substitution of control by intelligence for control by external authority, not the negative principle of no control or the spasmodic principle of control by emotional gusts, is the only basis upon which reformed education can build. To come into possession of intelligence is the sole human title to freedom. The spontaneity of childhood is a delightful and precious thing, but in its original naïve form it is bound to disappear. Emotions become sophisticated unless they become enlightened, and the manifestation of sophisticated emotion is in no sense genuine self-expression. True spontaneity is henceforth not a birth-right but the last term, the consummated conquest, of an art—the art of conscious control to the mastery of which Mr. Alexander's book so convincingly invites us.

## II

The principle and procedure set forth by Mr. Alexander are crucially needed at present. Strangely, this is the very reason why they are hard to understand and accept. For although there is nothing esoteric in his teaching, and although his exposition is made in the simplest English, free from technical words, it is difficult for anyone to grasp its full force without having actual demonstration of the principle in operation. And even then, as I know from personal experience, its full meaning dawns upon one only slowly and with new meanings continually opening up. Since I can add nothing to the clear and full exposition that Mr. Alexander has himself given, it has occurred to me that the most useful form this introductory word can take is an attempt to explain wherein lies the difficulty in grasping his principle.

The chief difficulty, as I have said, lies in the fact that it is so badly needed. The seeming contradiction in this statement is just one instance of the vicious circle which is frequently pointed out and fully dealt with in the pages of the text. The principle is badly needed, because in all matters that concern the individual self and the conduct of its life there is a defective and lowered sensory appreciation and judgment, both of ourselves and of our acts, which accompanies our wrongly-adjusted psychophysical mechanisms. It is precisely this perverted consciousness which we bring with us to the reading and comprehension of Mr. Alexander's pages, and which makes it hard for us to realize his statements as to its existence, causes, and effects. We have become so used to it that we take it for granted. It forms, as he has so clearly shown, our standard of rightness. It influences our every observation, interpretation, and judgment. It is the one factor which enters into our every act and thought.

Consequently, only when the results of Mr. Alexander's lessons have changed one's sensory appreciation and supplied a new standard, so that the old and the new condition can be compared with each other, does the concrete force of his teaching come home to one. In spite of the whole tenor of Mr. Alexander's teaching, it is this which makes it practically impossible for anyone to go to him with any other idea at the outset beyond that of gaining some specific relief and remedy. Even after a considerable degree of experience with his lessons, it is quite possible for one to prize his method merely on account of specific benefits received, even though one recognizes that these benefits include a changed emotional condition and a different outlook on life. Only when a pupil reaches the point of giving his full attention to the *method* of Mr. Alexander instead of its results, does he realize the constant influence of his sensory appreciation.

The perversion of our sensory consciousness of ourselves has gone so far that we lack criteria for judging the doctrines and methods that profess to deal with the individual human being. We oscillate between reliance upon plausible general theories and reliance upon testimonies to specific benefits obtained. We oscillate between extreme credulity and complete scepticism. On the one hand, there is the readiest acceptance of all claims made in behalf of panaceas when these are accompanied by testimonies of personal benefits and cures. On the other hand, the public has seen so many of these panaceas come and go that it has, quite properly, become sceptical about the reality of any new and different principle for developing human well-being. The world is flooded at present with various systems for relieving the ills that human flesh is heir to, such as systems of exercise for rectifying posture, methods of mental, psychological, and spiritual healing, so that, except when there happens to be an emotional wave sweeping the country, the very suggestion that there is fundamental truth in an unfamiliar principle is likely to call out the feeling that one more person, reasonably sensible about most things, has fallen for another one of the "cure-alls" that abound. "How," it will be asked, "can the teaching of Mr. Alexander be differentiated from these other systems? What assurance is there that it is anything more than one of them, working better perhaps for some persons and worse for others?" If, in reply, specific beneficial results of Mr. Alexander's teaching are pointed out, one is reminded of the fact that imposing testimonials of this kind can be produced in favor of all the other systems. The point, then, to be decided is: What is the worth of these results and how is their worth to be judged? Or, again, if it is a question of the theories behind the results, most of the systems are elaborately reasoned out and claim scientific or spiritual backing. In what fundamental respect, then, do the principles and consequences of Mr. Alexander's teaching differ from these?

These are fair questions, and it seems to me that probably the best thing that this introduction can do is to suggest some simple criteria by which any plan can be judged. Certain other questions may suggest the path by which these criteria may be found. Is a system primarily remedial, curative, aiming at relief of sufferings that already exist; or is it fundamentally preventive in nature? And if preventive rather than merely corrective, is it specific or general in scope? Does it deal with the "mind" and the "body" as things separated from each other, or does it deal with the unity of man's individuality? Does it deal with some portion or aspect of "mind" and "body" or with the re-education of the whole being? Does it aim at securing results directly, by treatment of symptoms, or does it deal with the *causes* of malconditions present in such a way that any beneficial results secured come as a natural consequence, almost, it might be said, as by-products of a fundamental change in such conditioning causes? Is the scheme educational or non-educational in character? If the principle underlying it claims to be preventive and constructive, does it operate from without by setting up some automatic safety-device, or does it operate from within? Is it cheap and easy, or does it make demands on the intellectual and moral energies of the individuals concerned? Unless it does the latter, what is it, after all, but a scheme depending ultimately upon some trick or magic, which, in curing one trouble, is sure to leave behind it other troubles (including fixations, inhibitions, laxities, lessening of power of steady and intelligent control), since it does not deal with causes, but only directs their operation into different channels, and changes symptoms from such as are perceptible into more subtle ones that are not perceived? Anyone who bears such questions as the above in mind whilst reading Mr. Alexander's book will have little difficulty in discriminating between the principles underlying his educational method and those of the systems with which it might be compared and confused.

Any sound plan must prove its soundness in reference both to concrete consequences and to general principles. What we too often forget is that these principles and facts must not be judged separately, but in connexion with each other. Further, whilst any theory or principle must ultimately be judged by its consequences in operation, whilst it must be verified experimentally by observation of how it works, yet in order to justify a claim to be scientific, it must provide a method for making evident and observable what the consequences are; and this method must be such as to afford a guarantee that the observed consequences actually flow from the principle. And I unhesitatingly assert that, when judged by this standard—that is, of a principle at work in effecting definite and verifiable consequences—Mr. Alexander's teaching is scientific in the strictest sense of the word. It meets both of these requirements. In other words, the plan of Mr. Alexander satisfies the most exacting demands of scientific method.

The principle or theory of Mr. Alexander and the observed consequences of its operation have developed at the same time and in the closest connexion with each other. Both have evolved out of an experimental method of procedure. At no time has he elaborated a theory for its own sake. This fact has occasionally been a disappointment to "intellectual" persons who have subconsciously got into the habit of depending upon a certain paraphernalia of technical terminology. But the theory has never been carried beyond the needs of the procedure employed, nor beyond experimentally verified results. Employing a remarkably sensitive power of observation, he has noted the actual changes brought about in individuals in response to the means which he has employed, and has followed up these changes in their connexions with the individual's habitual reflexes, noting the reactions due to the calling into play of established bad habits, with even greater care than the more obvious beneficial consequences obtained. Every such undesirable response has been treated as setting a problem—namely, that of discovering some method by which the evocation of these instinctive reactions, and the feelings associated with them, can be inhibited, and, in their stead, such acts called into play as will give a basis for correct sensory appreciations. Every step in the process has been analyzed and formulated, and every changing condition and consequence, positive or negative, favorable or unfavorable, which is employed as a means for developing the experimental procedure, has been still further developed. The use of this developed method has, of course, continuously afforded new material for observation and thorough analysis. To this process of simultaneous development of principles and consequences, used as means for testing each other, there is literally no end. As long as Mr. Alexander uses the method, it will be a process tending continually towards perfection. It will no more arrive at a stage of finished perfection than does any genuine experimental scientific procedure, with its theory and supporting facts. The most striking fact of Mr. Alexander's teaching is the sincerity and reserve with which he has never carried his formulation beyond the point of demonstrated facts.

It is obvious, accordingly, that the results obtained by Mr. Alexander's teaching stand on a totally different plane from those obtained under the various systems which have had great vogue until they have been displaced by some other tide of fashion and publicity. Most of those who urge the claims of these systems point to "cures" and other specific phenomena as evidence that they are built upon correct principles. Even for patent medicines an abundance of testimonials can be adduced. But the theories and the concrete facts in these cases have no genuine connexion with each other. Certain consequences, the "good" ones, are selected and held up for notice, whilst no attempt is made to find out what other consequences are taking place. The "good" ones are swallowed whole. There is no method by which it can be shown what consequences, if any, result from the principle invoked, or whether they are due to quite other causes.

But the essence of scientific method does not consist in taking consequences in gross; it consists precisely in the means by which consequences are followed up in detail. It consists in the processes by which the causes that are used to explain the consequences, or effects, can be concretely followed up to show that they actually produce these consequences and no others. If, for instance, a chemist pointed, on the one hand, to a lot of concrete phenomena which had occurred after he had tried an experiment and, on the other hand, to a lot of general principles and theories elaborately reasoned out, and then proceeded to assert that the two things were connected so that the theoretical principles accounted for the phenomena, he would meet only with ridicule. It would be clear that scientific method had not even been started; it would be clear that he was offering nothing but assertion.

Mr. Alexander has persistently discouraged the appeal to "cures" or to any other form of remarkable phenomena. He has even discouraged keeping records of these cases. Yet, if he had not been so wholeheartedly devoted to working out a demonstration

of a principle—a demonstration in the scientific sense of the word
—he would readily have had his day of vogue as one among the
miracle-mongers. He has also persistently held aloof from building
up an imposing show of technical scientific terminology of physiology, anatomy, and psychology. Yet that course also would have
been easy in itself, and a sure method of attracting a following.
As a consequence of this sincerity and thoroughness, maintained
in spite of great odds, without diversion to side-issues of fame and
external success, Mr. Alexander has demonstrated a new scientific
principle with respect to the control of human behaviour, as important as any principle which has ever been discovered in the
domain of external nature. Not only this, but his discovery is
necessary to complete the discoveries that have been made about
non-human nature, if these discoveries and inventions are not to
end by making us their servants and helpless tools.

A scientific man is quite aware that no matter how extensive
and thorough is his theoretical reasoning, and how definitely it
points to a particular conclusion of fact, he is not entitled to assert
the conclusion as a fact until he has actually observed the fact,
until his senses have been brought into play. With respect to dis-
tinctively human conduct, no one, before Mr. Alexander, has even
considered just what kind of sensory observation is needed in order
to test and work out theoretical principles. Much less have thinkers
in this field ever evolved a technique for bringing the requisite
sensory material under definite and usable control. Appeal to suggestion, to the unconscious and to the subconscious, is in its very
description an avoidance of this scientific task; the systems of
purely physical exercise have equally neglected any consideration
of the methods by which their faults are to be observed and
analyzed.

Whenever the need has been dimly felt for some concrete
check and realization of the meaning of our thoughts and judgments about ourselves and our conduct, we have fallen back, as
Mr. Alexander has so clearly pointed out in his writings, on our
pre-existing sense of what is "right." But this signifies in the concrete only what we feel to be *familiar*. And in so far as we have
bad habits needing re-education, that which is familiar in our sense
of ourselves and of our acts can only be a reflection of the bad

psycho-physical habits that are operating within us. This, of course, is precisely as if a scientific man, who, by a process of reasoning, had been led to a belief in what we call the Copernican theory, were then to try to test this reasoning by appealing to precisely those observations, without any addition or alteration, which had led men to the Ptolemaic theory. Scientific advance manifestly depends upon the discovery of conditions for making new observations, and upon the re-making of old observations under different conditions; in other words, upon methods of discovering *why,* as in the case of the scientific man, we have had and relied upon observations that have led into error.

After studying over a period of years Mr. Alexander's method in actual operation, I would stake myself upon the fact that he has applied to our ideas and beliefs about ourselves and about our acts exactly the same method of experimentation and of production of new sensory observations, as tests and means of developing thought, that have been the source of all progress in the physical sciences; and if, in any other plan, any such use has been made of the sensory appreciation of our attitudes and acts, if in it there has been developed a technique for creating new sensory observations of ourselves, and if complete reliance has been placed upon these findings, I have never heard of it. In some plans there has been a direct appeal to "consciousness" (which merely registers bad conditions); in some, this consciousness has been neglected entirely and dependence placed instead upon bodily exercises, rectifications of posture, etc. But Mr. Alexander has found a method for detecting precisely the correlations between these two members, physical-mental, of the same whole, and for creating a new sensory consciousness of new attitudes and habits. It is a discovery which makes whole all scientific discoveries, and renders them available, not for our undoing, but for human use in promoting our constructive growth and happiness.

No one would deny that we ourselves enter as an agency into whatever is attempted and done by us. That is a truism. But the hardest thing to attend to is that which is closest to ourselves, that which is most constant and familiar. And this closest "something" is, precisely, ourselves, our own habits and ways of doing things as agencies in conditioning what is tried or done by us. Through modern science we have mastered to a wonderful extent the use of things as tools for accomplishing results upon and through other things. The result is all but a universal state of confusion, discontent, and strife. The one factor which is the primary tool in the use of all these other tools—namely, ourselves—in other words, our own psycho-physical disposition, as the basic condition of our employment of all agencies and energies, has not even been studied as the central instrumentality. Is it not highly probable that this failure gives the explanation of why it is that in mastering physical forces we have ourselves been so largely mastered by them, until we find ourselves incompetent to direct the history and destiny of man?

Never before, I think, has there been such an acute consciousness of the failure of all external remedies as exists today, of the failure of all remedies and forces external to the individual man. It is, however, one thing to teach the need of a return to the individual man as the ultimate agency in whatever mankind and society collectively can accomplish, to point out the necessity of straightening out this ultimate condition of whatever humanity in mass can attain. It is another thing to discover the concrete procedure by which this greatest of all tasks can be executed. And this indispensable thing is exactly what Mr. Alexander has accomplished. The discovery could not have been made and the method of procedure perfected except by dealing with adults who were badly co-ordinated. But the method is not one of remedy; it is one of constructive education. Its proper field of application is with the young, with the growing generation, in order that they may come to possess as early as possible in life a correct standard of sensory appreciation and self-judgment. When once a reasonably adequate part of a new generation has become properly co-ordinated, we shall have assurance for the first time that men and women in the future will be able to stand on their own feet, equipped with satisfactory psycho-physical equilibrium, to meet with readiness, confidence, and happiness instead of with fear, confusion, and discontent, the buffetings and contingencies of their surroundings.

## III

In writing some introductory words to Mr. Alexander's previous book, *Constructive Conscious Control of the Individual*,

I stated that his procedure and conclusions meet all the requirements of the strictest scientific method, and that he has applied the method in a field in which it had never been used before—that of our judgments and beliefs concerning ourselves and our activities. In so doing, he has, I said in effect, rounded out the results of the sciences in the physical field, accomplishing this end in such a way that they become capable of use for human benefit. It is a commonplace that scientific technique has for its consequence control of the energies to which it refers. Physical science has for its fruit an astounding degree of new command of physical energies. Yet we are faced with a situation which is serious, perhaps tragically so. There is everywhere increasing doubt as to whether this physical mastery of physical energies is going to further human welfare, or whether human happiness is going to be wrecked by it. Ultimately there is but one sure way of answering this question in the hopeful and constructive sense. If there can be developed a technique which will enable individuals really to secure the right use of themselves, then the factor upon which depends the final use of all other forms of energy will be brought under control. Mr. Alexander has evolved this technique.

In repeating these statements, I do so fully aware of their sweeping nature. Were not our eyes and ears so accustomed to irresponsible statements that we cease to ask for either meaning or proof, they might well raise a question as to the complete intellectual responsibility and competency of their author. In repeating them after the lapse of intervening years, I appeal to the account which Mr. Alexander has given of the origin of his discovery of the principle of central and conscious control. Those who do not identify science with a parade of technical vocabulary will find in this account the essentials of scientific method in any field of inquiry. They will find a record of long continued, patient, unwearied experimentation and observation in which every inference is extended, tested, corrected by further more searching experiments; they will find a series of such observations in which the mind is carried from observation of comparatively coarse, gross, superficial connections of causes and effect to those causal conditions which are fundamental and central in the use which we make of ourselves.

Personally, I cannot speak with too much admiration—in the original sense of wonder as well as the sense of respect—of the persistence and thoroughness with which these extremely difficult observations and experiments were carried out. In consequence, Mr. Alexander created what may be truly called a physiology of the *living* organism. His observations and experiments have to do with the actual functioning of the body, with the organism in operation, and in operation under the ordinary conditions of living —rising, sitting, walking, standing, using arms, hands, voice, tools, instruments of all kinds. The contrast between sustained and accurate observations of the living and the usual activities of man and those made upon dead things under unusual and artificial conditions marks the difference between true and pseudo-science. And yet so used have we become to associating "science" with the latter sort of thing that its contrast with the genuinely scientific character of Mr. Alexander's observations has been one great reason for the failure of many to appreciate his technique and conclusions.

As might be anticipated, the conclusions of Mr. Alexander's experimental inquiries are in harmony with what physiologists know about the muscular and nervous structure. But they give a new significance to that knowledge; indeed, they make evident what knowledge itself really is. The anatomist may "know" the exact function of each muscle, and conversely know what muscles come into play in the execution of any specified act. But if he is himself unable to co-ordinate all the muscular structures involved in, say, sitting down or in rising from a sitting position in a way which achieves the optimum and efficient performance of that act; if, in other words, he misuses himself in what he does, how can he be said to *know* in the full and vital sense of that word? Magnus proved by means of what may be called *external* evidence the existence of a central control in the organism. But Mr. Alexander's technique gave a direct and intimate confirmation in personal experience of the fact of central control long before Magnus carried on his investigations. And one who has had experience of the technique *knows* it through the series of experiences which he himself has. The genuinely scientific character of Mr. Alexander's teaching and discoveries can be safely rested upon this fact alone.

The vitality of a scientific discovery is revealed and tested in its power to project and direct new further operations which not only harmonize with prior results but which lead on to new observed materials, suggesting in turn further experimentally controlled acts, and so on in a continued series of new developments. Speaking as a pupil, it was because of this fact as demonstrated in personal experience that I first became convinced of the scientific quality of Mr. Alexander's work. Each lesson was a laboratory experimental demonstration. Statements made in advance of consequences to follow and the means by which they would be reached were met with implicit scepticism—a fact which is practically inevitable, since, as Mr. Alexander points out, one uses the very conditions that need re-education as one's standard of judgment. Each lesson carries the process somewhat further and confirms in the most intimate and convincing fashion the claims that are made. As one goes on, new areas are opened, new possibilities are seen and then realized; one finds himself continually growing, and realizes that there is an endless process of growth initiated.

From one standpoint, I had an unusual opportunity for making an intellectual study of the technique and its results. I was, from the practical standpoint, an inept, awkward and slow pupil. There were no speedy and seemingly miraculous changes to evoke gratitude emotionally, while they misled me intellectually. I was forced to observe carefully at every step of the process, and to interest myself in the theory of the operations. I did this partly from my previous interest in psychology and philosophy, and partly as a compensation for my practical backwardness. In bringing to bear whatever knowledge I already possessed—or thought I did—and whatever powers of discipline in mental application I had acquired in the pursuit of these studies, I had the most humiliating experience of my life, intellectually speaking. For to find that one is unable to execute directions, including inhibitory ones, in doing such a seemingly simple act as to sit down, when one is using all the mental capacity which one prides himself upon possessing, is not an experience congenial to one's vanity. But it may be conducive to analytic study of causal conditions, obstructive and positive. And so I verified in personal experience all that Mr. Alexander says about the unity of the physical and psychical in the psychophysical; about our habitually wrong use of ourselves and the part this wrong use plays in generating all kinds of unnecessary tensions and wastes of energy; about the vitiation of our sensory appreciations which form the material of our judgments of ourselves; about the unconditional necessity of inhibition of customary acts, and the tremendous mental difficulty found in not "doing" something as soon as an habitual act is suggested, together with the great change in moral and mental attitude that takes place as proper co-ordinations are established. In re-affirming my conviction as to the scientific character of Mr. Alexander's discoveries and technique, I do so then not as one who has experienced a "cure," but as one who has brought whatever intellectual capacity he has to the study of a problem. In the study, I found the things which I had "known"—in the sense of theoretical belief—in philosophy and psychology, changed into vital experiences which gave a new meaning to knowledge of them.

In the present state of the world, it is evident that the control we have gained of physical energies, heat, light, electricity, etc., without having first secured control of our use of ourselves is a perilous affair. Without control of our use of ourselves, our use of other things is blind; it may lead to anything.

Moreover, if our habitual judgments of ourselves are warped because they are based on vitiated sense material—as they must be if our habits of managing ourselves are already wrong—then the more complex the social conditions under which we live, the more disastrous must be the outcome. Every additional complication of outward instrumentalities is likely to be a step nearer destruction: a fact which the present state of the world tragically exemplifies.

The school of Pavloff has made current the idea of conditioned reflexes. Mr. Alexander's work extends and corrects the idea. It proves that there are certain basic, central organic habits and attitudes which condition *every* act we perform, every use we make of ourselves. Hence a conditioned reflex is not just a matter of an arbitrarily established connection, such as that between the sound of a bell and the eating-reaction in a dog, but goes back to central conditions within the organism itself. This discovery corrects the ordinary conception of the conditioned reflex. The latter as usually understood renders an individual a passive puppet to be played upon by external manipulations. The discovery of a central control which conditions all other reactions brings the conditioning factor under conscious direction and enables the individual through his own co-ordinated activities to take possession of his own potentialities. It converts the fact of conditioned reflexes from a principle of external enslavement into a means of vital freedom.

Education is the only sure method which mankind possesses for directing its own course. But we have been involved in a vicious circle. Without knowledge of what constitutes a truly normal and healthy psycho-physical life, our professed education is likely to be mis-education. Every serious student of the formation of disposition and character which takes place in the family and school knows—speaking without the slightest exaggeration—how often and how deplorably this possibility is realized. The technique of Mr. Alexander gives to the educator a standard of psycho-physical health—in which what we call morality is included. It supplies also the "means whereby" this standard may be progressively and endlessly achieved, becoming a conscious possession of the one educated. It provides therefore the conditions for the central direction of all special educational processes. It bears the same relation to education that education itself bears to all other human activities.

I cannot therefore state too strongly the hopes that are aroused in me by the information contained in the Appendix that Mr. Alexander has, with his coadjutors, opened a training class, nor my sense of the importance that this work secures adequate support. It contains in my judgment the promise and potentiality of the new direction that is needed in all education.

# PREFACE TO BOOK BY ALEXANDER

by George E. Coghill

The practice of Mr. F. Matthias Alexander in treating the human body is founded, as I understand it, on three well-established biological principles, 1) that of the integration of the whole organism in the performance of particular functions, 2) that of proprioceptive sensitivity as a factor in determining posture, 3) that of the primary importance of posture in determining muscular action. These principles I have established through forty years of anatomical and physiological study of Amblystoma of embryonic and larval stages, and they appear to hold for other vertebrates as well.

In order to make this discussion clear, definitions of certain terms are necessary. Normally, as regards somatic (general bodily) motor function, the organism exists in a condition of mobility or immobility—either as mobilized or as immobilized. The latter condition is illustrated by sleep. In deep sleep the individual is mobilized in regard to its visceral, circular and respiratory functions and the like, but it is immobilized with reference to bodily movement. Reflexes occur, to be sure, to local stimuli, but as an individual the body as a whole does nothing for its own sake. Somnambulism, as a general bodily activity, occurs during periods of imperfect sleep or partial wakefulness. In the condition of immobility the individual may be thought of as in repose. In mobility, on the other hand, the whole individual is mobilized (integrated), or in action as a unit according to a definite pattern. Under these circumstances the organism is in one of two phases of action, posture or movement. Posture is relatively static in so far as the individual as a whole is concerned; movement is transition through space for the organism or its parts. In posture the individual is mobilized for a definite movement in which the energy mobilized in posture is released in a definite pattern of activity. Of course these differences are relative, and one phase passes over imperceptibly into the other, but in their typical manifestations they are clearly differentiated. Likewise the distinction between mobility and immobility is relative, and no absolute distinction can be made between them, but the distinction is useful if not necessary for a clear understanding of physiological principles. It seems reasonable, therefore, to propose that in posture the individual is mobilized (integrated) for movement according to a definite pattern and in movement that pattern is being executed. In posture the individual is as truly active as in movement.

Another term that may need explanation is "proprioceptive," which applies to sensory nerves that serve the muscles, tendons and joints, and the middle ear (vestibular apparatus) and its nerves. The proprioceptive system has nothing to do with local or cutaneous sensation.

Mr. Alexander has found these same principles operative also in man. His work is concerned with the nature of the influence of the working of the psycho-physical mechanisms upon the general functioning of the human organism (posture), and his technique was evolved as an aid in maintaining the general conditions best suited to this working in those in whom they already exist, and in changing and improving them when this working can be shown to be harmful. He has further demonstrated the very important psychological principle that the proprioceptive system can be brought under conscious control, and can be educated to carry to the motor centers the stimulus which is responsible for the muscular activity which brings about the manner of working (use) of the mechanism of correct posture. Of course the time required for this education could be greatly lessened through the assistance of a competent teacher.

To understand the first biological principle mentioned, the relation of the part to the whole, it is necessary to know this relation in the development of behavior, which I have investigated for many years. My studies have been both anatomical and physiological, those of the one method corroborating, supplementing and extending those of the other. For these investigations I used a species of Amblystoma, a type of vertebrate that is well known for its lack of specialization of structure and function and in which movement can be observed under controlled conditions from the first. Like the other Amphibia, it is both terrestrial and aquatic so that the development of locomotion by both swimming and walking can be studied.

In these animals at the time muscular contraction begins the whole functional muscular system is organized as to longitudinal bilateral series of segment, the myotomes. At that time there are no appendages other than relatively homogeneous buds composed of undifferentiated tissue covered with skin. These are not functional organs, and will not be for a relatively long time after the motility of the trunk musculature begins. When the axial muscles begin to contract their contraction proceeds from the head tailward (cephalocaudal). If the stimulus is adequate the whole animal responds as a total reaction. There is never a partial response in the sense of a local reaction except in the anterior end where contraction of a few myotomes may occur in case the stimulus is not adequate to stimulate the entire system, for the organization is such that a stimulus arising anywhere on the trunk or tail must travel headward in the dorsal part of the spinal cord in order to reach the motor centers. Also the motor neurones are integrating neurones of the axial muscles, that is to say, they are at the same time longitudinal conductors in the spinal cord and motor nerves, innervating the muscles simply by means of collateral (side branches of the axones). These collaterals grow out into the limbs and establish a functional connection with the muscles of the limbs so that the earliest movements of the limbs are performed only as the trunk moves. The limbs are therefore primarily integrated with the trunk, and local reflexes do not occur. These are made possible through another type of neurones, which arise from a different source in the spinal cord from the integrating neurones that give rise to the primary motor fibers. There are, therefore, two possible functions of the limbs: a primary one wholly and always integrated with the trunk, and a secondary one in response to local stimuli. The first gives rise to total reactions and the latter elicits reflexes, and reflexes as partial pattern are normally always subject to the total pattern.

1 The principles derived by Coghill from his study of these salamanders have been extended by subsequent research to human fetuses (Davenport Hooker, Tryphena Humphrey).

In the course of development of behavior of Amblystoma the earliest partial reactions are postural. If, for example, one can succeed in rolling the animal over from the upright to the supine position by means of a bristle without exciting it to other action, one leg will be elevated and the opposite one depressed in the turning process. The movement has the appearance of a local reaction (partial pattern) but it is not in response to a local stimulus from the skin. It is in response to stimuli arising in the proprioceptive system. There are two possible sources of proprioceptive stimulation. In the first place there are sensory endings in the axial muscles of the earliest reaction stages, and the forced torsion of the axial muscles would stimulate these proprioceptive nerves and they could stimulate the elevation and depression of the limbs. As a second possibility the vestibular system of the ear is sufficiently developed to be functional at this stage of development, and long fibers from the vestibular centers in the brain travel far down the spinal cord and into the motor centers that innervate the limbs. Whether one or both of these sensory systems are responsible for these postural reactions of the limbs it is the animal as a whole that stimulates the response. The earliest postural reaction of the limbs, therefore, is a total reaction, and the sensory factor is in the proprioceptive system. The stimuli arise wholly within the organism.

In the development of Amblystoma I have observed, also, that an appropriate posture is assumed at intervals for an appreciable time before the particular muscular pattern is geared to action. This occurs in the development of swimming, of walking and of feeding. Posture, therefore, is a forerunner of action and must be regarded as basic to it.

These are the simple rudiments of movement which Mr. Alexander calls into play by his methods of reeducation. For he is pre-eminently an educator. He seeks to restore the functions of the body through their natural uses. His methods of doing this are original and unique, based, as they are, on many years of experience and exhaustive study. Yet they can scarcely be adequately described, although the results are marvelous.

One ordinarily considers that rising from a sitting position in a chair to a standing position is a simple process perfectly understood by every adult. But this pattern of behavior is not natural.

It was introduced into our behavior very late in our racial development with the invention of the chair, the most atrocious institution hygienically of civilized life. Primitive man sat on the ground or squatted when not standing. Primitive man does so still, and the ease and apparent comfort of the squatting position is witnessed among the less privileged classes, who rest in that position for long periods. This posture requires extreme stretching of the extensor muscles of the legs and abduction of the thighs. Habitual use of the chair, on the other hand, prevents this stretching of the extensor muscles and tends to produce adduction of the thighs, even to the extreme of crossing one leg over the other. This unnatural posture tends to stimulate reflex responses which antagonize the normal total pattern of rising to a standing position.

That this is more than theory Mr. Alexander demonstrated to me in lessons which he kindly gave me. He enabled me to prevent misdirection of the muscles of my neck and back and to bring about a use of these muscles that determined the relative position of my head and neck to my body and so on to my limbs, bringing my thighs into the abducted position. This led to changes in the muscular and other conditions throughout my body and limbs associated with a pattern of behavior more natural (in agreement with the total pattern) for the act of getting on my feet. The whole procedure was calculated to occupy my brain with the projection of directive messages that would enable me to acquire conscious control of the proprioceptive component of the reflex mechanism involved. The projection of the directed messages, Mr. Alexander considers, stimulated nervous and motor activity that was associated with better conditions. This leads to the belief that the motor paths of the spinal cord and the nerve paths through the brain associated with the total pattern were again being used.

In my study of the development of locomotion I have found that in vertebrates the locomotor function involves two patterns: a total pattern which establishes the gait; and partial patterns (reflexes) which act with reference to the surface on which locomotion occurs. The sloth, for instance, has the same total pattern (gait) of walking that the dog has but employs a wholly different partial pattern (reflexes) for he supports himself in suspension with his flexor muscles. Now the reflexes may be, and naturally are, in harmony with the total pattern, in which case they facilitate the mechanism of the total pattern (gait), or they by force of habit become more or less antagonistic to it. In the latter case they make for inefficiency in locomotion. In myself, for example, when I have given attention to details of walking, I have experienced flexion of my toes as if they were trying to grasp the soles of my shoes. This I regard as a reflex brought about by habitual incorrect posture, and antagonistic to the natural gait which my toes, nevertheless, were trying to reinforce.

It is my opinion that habitual use of improper reflex mechanism in sitting, standing, and walking introduces conflict in the nervous system, and that this conflict is the cause of fatigue and nervous strain which bring many ills in their train. Mr. Alexander, by relieving this conflict between the total pattern which is hereditary and innate, and the reflex mechanisms which are individually cultivated, conserves the energies of the nervous system and by so doing corrects not only postural difficulties but also many other pathological conditions that are not ordinarily recognized as postural. This is a corrective principle that the individual learns for himself and is the work of the self as a whole. It is not a system of physical culture which involves only one system of organs for better or for worse of the economy of the whole organism. Mr. Alexander's method lays hold of the individual as a whole, as a self-vitalizing agent. He reconditions and reeducates the reflex mechanisms and brings their habits into normal relation with the functions of organisms as a whole. I regard his methods as thoroughly scientific and educationally sound.

# METHOD FOR CHANGING STEREOTYPED RESPONSE PATTERNS BY THE INHIBITION OF POSTURAL SETS

by Frank Pierce Jones

## ANATOMICAL MECHANISMS

The head can be rotated, tilted, or lowered by contracting the muscles attached to it; but it cannot be lifted. It can be lifted only by straightening and lengthening the cervical spine. Between the vertebrae and the skin there are four structures whose joint action determines the height of the head and its angle of tilt and rotation. They are shown schematically in Figure 1.

### Intervertebral Discs

The cartilaginous discs between the bodies of the vertebrae contain fluid and are capable of exerting hydraulic force on the bony structures around them (Gray, 1942, p. 281). The discs are kept under pressure by ligaments and by various muscles, including the small muscles which run from one vertebra to the next. If these muscles shorten, the distance between the vertebral bodies will be lessened, and the discs will be further compressed. Conversely, if they lengthen, the distance will increase as a result of the released pressure of the discs. In the intervertebral discs, then, is a mechanism by which the height of the head can be altered a small but significant amount.

### Flexors and Extensors of the Neck

Both convexity (extension) of the cervical curve and its forward inclination (flexion) are countered by the tension of ligaments and muscles whose origins and insertions are on the vertebrae themselves (Gray, 1942, pp. 390, 394–395). Acting together,

191

the flexors and extensors of the neck straighten and strengthen the cervical spine, turning it into a column of support and, in so doing, increase the height of the head.[1]

### Flexors and Extensors of the Head: I

In the upright posture, the head is in unstable equilibrium, its center of gravity forward of the base of support (the atlas), and its weight balanced by the tension of ligaments and muscles which run from insertion points at the base of the skull to various origins along the spinal column. These muscles, the extensors of the head, are designed to balance, in addition to the weight of the head, the tension in a smaller group of flexor muscles in front. By the lengthening and shortening of the various muscles in these two groups the head can be moved in many directions without destroying the equilibrium of forces (Gray, 1942, pp. 386–395).

### Flexors and Extensors of the Head: II. Sternomastoid and Upper Trapezius

There are two pairs of flexors and extensors which connect the head directly with the shoulder girdle. They are the *sternocleido-mastoids* (Gray, 1942, p. 384) and the *upper trapezii,* which form a blunted isosceles triangle at the back of the neck (Gray, 1942, p. 428). Simultaneous contraction of the two pairs of muscles will bring the head closer to the shoulder girdle and increase the curve of the cervical spine, the sternomastoid drawing the head forward and down, the *upper trapezius* preventing forward rotation by re-

[1] In standard textbooks of anatomy, the extensors of the head and the extensors of the neck are treated under a single heading and illustrated with the same plates so that it is sometimes difficult to distinguish one group of muscles from the other. They have similar names (*splenius, longissimus,* etc.) and similar origins on the spinal column. They differ, however, in their insertions and in the functions which they perform. When the neck is flexed, the head is brought forward and down. If, then, the neck extensors contract, the spine will be straightened (extended), and in the process the head will be brought to a higher level, even though the head extensors remain relaxed. Contracting the head extensors, on the other hand, will not lift the head, but will only tilt it backward so that the occiput approaches the seventh cervical vertebra. Duchenne (1959, p. 534) first pointed out in 1867 the difference of function between the two sets of extensor muscles. He had observed that patients whose neck extensors were paralyzed could not lift their heads, though they still had the full use of their head extensors.

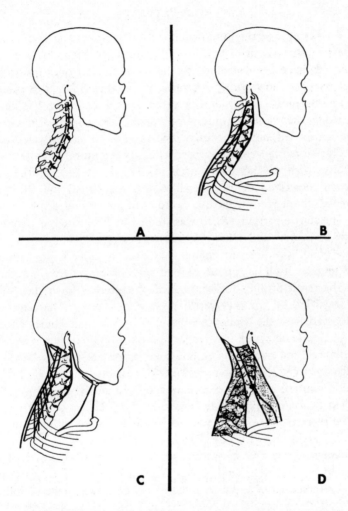

FIG. 1. Anatomical structures affecting the height and angle of the head. (A, intervertebral disks with *interspinales* and *intertransversarii* muscles. B, flexors and extensors of the neck. C, flexors and extensors of the head. D, *upper trapezius* and *sternocleido-mastoid* muscles.)

tracting the occiput.[1] In the process, the origins and insertions of the muscles and ligaments which maintain the weight of the head against gravity will be brought closer together.

## STARTLE PATTERN

An example of the joint action of the *sternomastoid* and *upper trapezius* can be seen in the "startle pattern" of Figure 2. Surface electrodes have been attached to the subject's skin over the right *sternomastoid* and right *upper trapezius*. In Figure 2A he is standing in his "most comfortable posture." In Figure 2B he has been startled by the sudden slamming of a door. The two sets of muscles have contracted simultaneously. The head is thrust forward, but the Frankfort plane remains horizontal. The postural change does not stop with the head and neck. As in one of the "attitudinal reflexes" described below, the shoulders are lifted, the chest is flattened, the legs are flexed, and the arms are extended.

The startle pattern, which was studied with high-speed photography by Landis and Hunt (1939), provides a vivid example of how "good" posture can change to "bad" in a very brief time. The pattern itself is typical of bad posture in general, whether it is the result of age, disease, or lack of exercise (Jones, Hanson, & Gray, 1964). In the startle pattern, the active character of malposture and the sequence of events by which it comes about can be clearly observed. The response is not instantaneous. It begins in the head and neck, passing down the trunk and legs to be completed in about ½ second. The neck muscles are central in the organization of the response. Jones and Kennedy (1951), who studied the startle pattern by multiple-channel electromyography, placed surface electrodes in various locations on the subject's neck, trunk, and limbs, with one pair always over the *upper trapezius*. The intensity of the stimulus was varied from the sound of a dropped book to the sound of a .32 caliber revolver. Sixty patterns were obtained from eight subjects. In all cases when the stimulus

---

[1] It may be significant that the two muscles have the same phylogenetic origin (Romer, 1949, p. 285) and that, unlike other neck muscles, they receive their principal innervation from a cranial nerve (the accessory). Duchenne (1959, p. 5) commented on their extreme sensitivity to electrical stimulation, which he attributed to the peculiar character of their nerve supply.

was strong enough to elicit a response, it appeared in the neck muscles; in many cases, the response appeared nowhere else.

## PHYSIOLOGICAL MECHANISMS

I have described two reciprocal sets of structures in the neck, one designed to straighten the cervical spine and move the head out from the trunk, the other designed to bring head and trunk closer together and increase the spinal curvature. In the procedure described earlier in this paper,[1] the downward pull of the *sternomastoid* and *upper trapezius* was counterbalanced by the experimenter while the subject moved. It is conjectured that in the process, the pressure on the discs was reduced, the flexors and extensors of the neck shortened, and a lengthening took place in the flexors and extensors of the head and in the small muscles between the vertebrae. During movement, the lengthening which appeared in the neck could be expected by purely mechanical means to extend along the rest of the spine, with the force being transmitted by muscle and ligament from one vertebra to the next.

### Stretch Reflexes

The mechanical effect of stretch on muscle is modified by the action of the nervous system. When a muscle is stretched, it contracts reflexly, and the strength of the contraction is proportional to the stretch. Though stretch reflexes occur at the spinal level, they are under the influence of higher centers in the nervous system. This influence is transmitted directly to the muscles through the system of small motoneurons, the gamma efferents. As the level of activity in the gamma efferents rises or falls, the sensitivity of a muscle to stretch increases or decreases. Whether a contracting muscle shortens or lengthens (as in lowering a weight), the stretch reflex persists as long as the stretch stimulus is applied. Though the range of lengths over which muscles can contract is considerable, there is an optimal "resting length" at which a particular muscle exerts maximum tension.

It seems reasonable to suppose that one effect of the experimental procedures is to reorganize stretch reflexes in the neck and

---

[1] An experimental version of the technique.

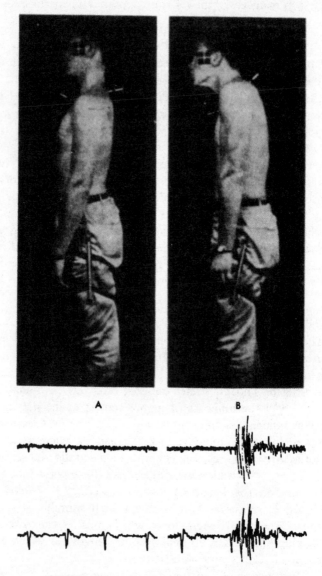

FIG. 2. Activity of neck muscles in the startle pattern. (A, subject standing in "most comfortable posture." B, subject after door slam. EMG records: above —*upper trapezius;* below—*sternomastoid.*)

back so that more muscle fibers take part in the antigravity response, and that the muscles in contracting remain closer to their optimal resting length. This effect would account for the subjective feeling of reduced weight while maintaining a position, as well as for the apparent lack of effort in movements performed against gravity.

### Head-Neck Reflexes

The kinesthetic phenomenon and the change in the movement pattern cannot be explained entirely by the behavior of individual muscles. Such an explanation does not account for the major role which the head and neck appear to play in facilitating the movement, nor for the secondary changes, e.g., in breathing, reported by subjects.

In the posture of animals, it is well established that the most important mechanism of control is the head-neck relation. Magnus and his associates (Magnus, 1924; Magnus & de Kleijn, 1912; Rademaker, 1931), in a long series of carefully controlled experiments, showed that the position of an animal's head in space or its position relative to the body can affect the distribution of tonus in its neck, back, and limbs. Magnus summed up the principle by saying that in posture and movement the head leads and the body follows.

In classifying his material, Magnus used two categories—the "attitudinal reflexes" and the "righting reflexes."

The *attitudinal* reflexes with receptors in the labyrinths and in the joints of the neck (McCouch, Deering, & Ling, 1951) are used by an animal to maintain a position that is assumed for some special purpose, like that of a cat drinking from a saucer or looking up at a piece of meat held high. The position taken by the head imposes on the rest of the body an attitude which is maintained as long as it is functional. These attitudes are quite stereotyped and follow regular rules. According to Magnus, they are the most enduring and untiring of reflexes.

The *righting* reflexes take over when an animal is ready to return to the normal upright posture. The fixed position of the head is released; the imbalance of parts, registering at a postural center in the brain, initiates the righting response; as in the attitudinal reflexes, the head leads and the body follows. The mechanism is most strikingly demonstrated when a cat is held on its back in the air and then dropped. The instant it is let go it begins to right itself. The head turns first. As it turns, the tensions in the neck, back, and limbs are progressively altered. The body is twisted around, and the cat lands on its feet. (Marey's photographs of the phenomenon are reproduced by Chatfield, 1957, p. 205.)

Secondary effects of the head-neck reflexes on respiration, circulation, and eye position have also been demonstrated. In diving birds and mammals there is a highly developed set of reflexes which stops breathing and slows down the heart in order to conserve oxygen (Irving, 1939; Scholander, 1963). In ducks, this reflex is strongly reinforced by the change in the relation of head, neck, and body that takes place in diving. Huxley (1913) found that without immersing a duck in water, breathing could be stopped by bringing the head and neck into the diving position or by placing the duck on its back and dorsiflexing the head. Conversely, breathing was at once restored if the head was brought back to the normal posture. A similar postural mechanism to stop breathing and slow the heart was later demonstrated in diving mammals (Koppányi, 1929). A. de Kleijn (1920) used monkeys to demonstrate the effect of head-neck reflexes on the position of the eye in the orbit. He showed that the eyes moved down when the head was dorsiflexed and up when it was ventriflexed, and that the same shift in eye position took place when the head remained fixed and the trunk was rotated so as to bring the back closer to the occiput or the chest closer to the chin.

### Head-Neck Reflexes in Man

In human beings, the influence of the head-neck reflexes is masked by patterns of voluntary activity. The mechanisms are clearly present, however. They have been frequently demonstrated in infants (Gesell, 1954; Peiper, 1963), young children (Landau, 1923; Schaltenbrand, 1925), patients with neurological diseases

---

[1] The secondary effect of differences in the trunk-to-head relation on the position of the eyes, which was demonstrated in monkeys by de Kleijn (1920), was demonstrated in human infants by Voss (1927).

(Simons, 1923; Walshe, 1923), and in normal adults (Hellebrandt, Schade, & Cairns, 1962; Tokizane, 1951; Wells, 1944). A large number of drawings and photographs to illustrate the patterns of head-neck reflexes as they manifest themselves in dancing, sport, and everyday activity were brought together by Fukuda (1957).

Various specific reflexes, both attitudinal and righting, have been defined in the literature. Rather than describe them in detail, I should like here to emphasize what each set of reflexes has in common. In the attitudinal reflexes, the head is drawn into a fixed position and tonus is redistributed in the trunk and limbs. In the righting reflexes, again under the influence of the head, the normal distribution of tonus is restored. These two mechanisms will account most economically for the phenomena which have been described in this paper. The sitting or standing posture of the average person functions like an "attitude" which has been imposed on the body by the head. The procedures employed in the experimental movements, by releasing the head from its habitual attitude, facilitate the righting reflexes and bring the subject into a different orientation within the gravitational field. The changes in breathing, in circulation, and in the use of the eyes, which are sometimes reported, take place automatically by reflex facilitation when the head moves into its new relationship to the trunk.

## PSYCHOLOGICAL CONSIDERATIONS

I have described a mechanism by which the antigravity response can be facilitated. It is a mechanism which ordinarily operates below the level of consciousness. Magnus was emphatic that the righting reflexes are subcortical and inaccessible to direct conscious control.[1] An indirect control can be established, however, if the subject learns to recognize and inhibit maladaptive postural sets which interfere with the response of the organism to gravity.

In the course of motor learning, sets may be developed which

[1] Magnus (1925):

It seems to be of the greatest importance that the whole central apparatus for the righting function (with the only exception of the optical righting reflexes) is placed subcortically in the brain stem and by this means withdrawn from voluntary action. The cortex cerebri evokes during ordinary life a succession of phasic movements, which tend to *disturb* the normal resting posture. The brain-stem centres will in the meantime *restore* the disturbance and bring the body back into the normal posture, are not the best preparation for the movement to come. They may, in fact, hamper the execution of the movement. Unfortunately, like some of the "superstitious" responses which appear during conditioning experiments, such sets do not extinguish readily. The organism adapts to them quickly; they come to "feel right"; and they remain undetected, because once the stimulus to move has been received, attention becomes focused on the goal to be reached.

One of these inappropriate sets is the tendency to shorten neck muscles as a preparation for a movement against gravity. It has been demonstrated that such a movement is facilitated when the preparatory shortening of muscles is prevented by the experimenter. If the subject becomes aware of the tendency, he can learn to prevent it and thus establish an indirect control over the postural mechanism. In my experience, the only satisfactory way to achieve such a control is to reorganize the field of attention, so that when a stimulus to move is received, the focus of attention remains within the organism. This does not mean that the goal is excluded from attention; it means that the goal is not allowed to dominate the field. Attention is organized around the head-trunk relation, with extension in time and space so that both the stimulus and the response can be comprised within the same field.

Ordinarily, attention is directed either outward to the environment or inward to the organism itself. The central nervous system, however, is receiving information about movements and positions of the body and its parts at the same time that it receives information about events in the world outside. There is no reason why the field of attention cannot be organized in the same way. In such a field, the relation of the head, neck, and trunk, kinesthetically perceived, forms the background against which events outside and inside the organism take place. Thus it is possible to perceive an object simultaneously with the organism's reaction to it, since both are comprised within the same field.

Perceptually, objects are known to vary with the psychological context in which they are perceived. A staircase, for example, is per-

so that the next cortical impulse will find the body prepared to start again [p. 349].
  Magnus (1930):
  We have . . . a subcortically acting apparatus which controls and adjusts the position of our body, whether erect or recumbent, in relation to space. This unconsciously acting mechanism, by the cooperation of complicated reflexes, restores our body to the normal position whenever it is displaced [p. 103].

ceived differently depending on whether it is to be climbed or merely to be looked at. The difference, of course, lies within the perceiving organism. If it is a staircase to be climbed, it may elicit a postural set which is so marked that it can be detected by an outside observer. The set can be detected by the climber himself only if he reorganizes his field of attention so as to take in both the staircase and his reaction to it as he approaches and climbs it. With this shift in the focus of attention, he can perceive the cause-and-effect relation between the stimulus (the staircase) and his immediate response (the postural set). If he takes an experimental approach, he can devise a means to inhibit the set while continuing to make the specific response (climbing the stairs). In the process, the antigravity response will be facilitated in the same way as in the guided movements which were described above.

Climbing a staircase was used to illustrate a principle. Any activity—reaching for a pencil or making a speech—would have done as well. The principle of inhibition can be applied to any movement. A movement pattern is a complex whole which, for convenience, may be thought of as having two aspects or parts: a specific, goal-directed part, and a tonic or postural part, by which the integrity of the organism is maintained while the specific response is being carried out. The tonic or postural part of a movement is not ordinarily perceived. Tensional patterns which interfere with the smooth performance of movement can be perceived, however. If they are inhibited, postural tonus is redistributed, and the specific, goal-directed response becomes easier. In contrast to the ease of the facilitated movement, old ways of moving come to feel wrong, and a new sensory standard is gradually established.

In the paradigm of postural change which I have just outlined, inhibition is the basic principle. Inhibition is a term which has been used by psychologists and physiologists in a variety of meanings (Diamond, Balvin, & Diamond, 1963). I have used it here to describe a process by which a person consciously refrains from making a response which he could make if he chose. In this sense inhibition is the central function of

*a nervous system which, when it functions well, is able to exclude maladaptive conflict without suppressing spontaneity* [Diamond et al., p. 395].

In the presence of inhibition, a stimulus should elicit only a general-ized increase of alertness, leaving the organism free to respond or not respond.

The principle of inhibition, as it has been developed here, offers a new approach to the problem of behavioral change. In the close connection between inhibition and postural tonus is a mechanism which not only reveals the inner pattern of a stereotyped response but brings it under conscious control. In so doing, it greatly en-larges the area of behavior where free choice can operate.

# REFERENCES

CHATFIELD, P.O. "Fundamentals of clinical neurophysiology." Spring-field, Ill.: Charles C. Thomas, 1957.

DE KLEIJN, A. On the effect of tonic labyrinthine and cervical reflexes upon the eye muscles. "Koninklyke Akademie van Wetenschappen, Amsterdam Proceedings," 1920, 23, 509.

DIAMOND, S., BALVIN, R. S., & DIAMOND, F. R. "Inhibition and choice." New York: Harper & Row, 1963.

DUC. 'ENNE, G. B. "Physiologie des mouvements." (Orig. publ. 1867) (Physiology of Motion.) (Trans. by E. B. Kaplan) Philadelphia: W. B. Saunders, 1959.

FUKUDA, T. "Stato-kinetic reflexes in equilibrium and movement." Tokyo: Igaku Shoin, 1957.

GESELL, A. The ontogenesis of infant behavior. In L. Carmichael (ED.), "Manual of child psychology." New York: Wiley, 1954. Pp. 335–373.

GRAY, H. "Anatomy of the human body," (24th ed.) Philadelphia: Lea & Febiger, 1942.

HELLEBRANDT, FRANCES A., SCHADE, MAJA, & CAIRNS, MARIE L. Methods of evoking tonic neck reflexes in normal human subjects. "American Journal of Physical Medicine," 1962, 41, 90–139.

HUXLEY, FRANCES M. On the reflex nature of apnoea in the duck in diving. "Quarterly Journal of Experimental Physiology," 1913, 6, 147–196.

IRVING, L. Respiration in diving mammals. "Physiological Review," 1939, 19, 112–134.

JONES, F. P., HANSON, J. A., & GRAY, FLORENCE E. Startle as a paradigm of malposture. "Perceptual and Motor Skills," 1964, 19, 21–22.

JONES F. P., & KENNEDY, J. L. An electromyographic technique for recording the startle pattern. "Journal of Psychology," 1951, 32, 63–68.

KOPPANYI, T., & DOOLEY, M. S. Submergence and postural apnea in the muskrat. "American Journal of Physiology," 1929, 88, 592–595.

LANDAU, A. Über einen tonischen Lagereflex beim älteren Säugling. "Klinische Wochenschrift," 1923, 2, 1253–1255.

LANDIS, C., & HUNT, W. "The startle pattern." New York: Farrar & Rinehart, 1939.

McCOUCH, G. P., DEERING, I. D., & LING, T. H. Location of receptors for tonic neck reflexes. "Journal of Neurophysiology," 1951, 14, 191–195.

MAGNUS, R. "Korperstellung." Berlin: Springer, 1924.

MAGNUS, R. & DE KLEIJN, A. Die Abhängigkeit des Tonus der Extremitätenmuskeln von der Kopfstellung. "Pfügers Archiv für die gesamte Physiologie der Menschen und der Tiere," 1912, 145, 455–548.

PEIPER, A. Reflexes of position and movement. In, "Cerebral function in infancy and childhood." (Trans. by B. Nagler & Hilde Nagler) New York: Consultants Bureau, 1963, Ch. 4.

RADEMAKER, G. G. J. "Das Stehen." Berlin: Springer, 1931.

ROMER, A. S. "The vertebrate body." Philadelphia: W. B. Saunders, 1949.

SCHALTENBRAND, G. Normale Bewegungs- und Haltungs- und Lagereaktionen bei Kindern. "Deutsche Zeitschrift für Nervenheilkunde," 1925, 87, 23–42.

SCHOLANDER, P. F. The master switch of life. "Scientific American," 1963, 209, 92–106.

SIMONS, A. Kopfhaltung und Muskeltonus. "Zeitschrift für die gesamte Neurologie und Psychiatrie," 1923, 80, 499–549.

TOKIZANE, T., MURAO, M., OGATA, T., & KONDO, T. Electromyographic studies on tonic neck, lumbar and labyrinthine reflexes in normal persons. "Japanese Journal of Physiology," 1951, 2, 130–146.

VOSS, O. Geburtstrauma und Gehörorgan. "Acta oto-laryngologica," 1927, 11, 73–108.

WALSHE, F. M. R. On certain tonic or postural reflexes in hemiplegia with special reference to the so-called associated movements. "Brain," 1923, 46, 1–37.

WELLS, H. S. The demonstration of tonic neck and labyrinthine reflexes and positive heliotropic responses in normal human subjects. "Science," 1944, 99, 36–37.

(*abridged from* PSYCHOLOGICAL REVIEW, Vol. 72, No. 3, May, 1965)

## LEARNING BY YOURSELF

People have frequently introduced themselves to me with the statement: "I have read Mr. Alexander's books and I always try to hold my head in the right position, which he advocates." This, of course, is just what he did not advocate. He discovered an inhibitory control which has nothing to do with position. This was not an idle chance discovery. It followed a series of careful observations of the way he responded to the stress of public recitation. If you wanted to establish a similar control without expert assistance, you could design a few simple experiments in which you could subject yourself to mild stress and observe its effect on the muscles of your neck. For instance, if you lie down on your back and anticipate the effort you would make in order to sit up, you may detect an increase in tension in your neck even before you begin to move. See if you can inhibit this increase as you continue to think of sitting up but don't sit up. Then decide not to sit up but bring your right knee up while you inhibit the increase in neck-muscle tension. (Note that you are not relaxing tension that is already there but inhibiting an increase in response to the thought of raising your knee.) You may judge your success in two ways: (1) by how well you sustain your resolution to inhibit and (2) by the movement of the knee, which should follow a different pathway from the one it would ordinarily follow.

Another experimental situation you might devise would be to expose yourself to a disagreeable sound like an alarm clock or a piece of squeaking chalk, or merely to think of such a sound, and to observe in as much detail as possible how your body responded, giving special attention to the response of your head and neck. After obtaining a fairly clear perception of the pattern of your response, you could then experiment by inhibiting the change in level of neck-muscle tension and observing any changes that might take place in the rest of the response pattern. (*Body Awareness in Action,* p. 160, Schocken Books, 1976.)